MW01017362

CARING FOR PEOPLE WITH HIV

This book is especially dedicated to patients infected with HIV, their partners, families and friends affected by HIV and all professional and non-professional carers who support them.

Caring for People with HIV
A community perspective

Dr Surinder Singh
Department of Primary Care and Population Sciences
Royal Free Hospital School of Medicine

and

Dr Sara Madge
Department of HIV/AIDS
Royal Free Hospital Trust

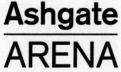

Ashgate
ARENA
Aldershot • Brookfield USA • Singapore • Sydney

© Surinder Singh and Sara Madge 1998

All rights reserved. No part of this publication may be reproduced, stored in a retrieval system, or transmitted in any form or by any means electronic, mechanical, photocopying, recording or otherwise without the prior permission of the publisher.

Published by
Ashgate Publishing Limited
Gower House
Croft Road
Aldershot
Hants GU11 3HR
England

Ashgate Publishing Company
Old Post Road
Brookfield
Vermont 05036
USA

British Library Cataloguing in Publication Data
Singh, Surinder
    Caring for people with HIV: a community perspective. –
(Social work)
    1. HIV infections 2. HIV-positive persons – Care
    I. Title   II. Madge, Sara
    362.1'969792

Library of Congress Catalog Card Number: 98–70993

ISBN (HBK) 1 85742 397 6
ISBN (PBK)   1 85742 398 4

Printed and bound in Great Britain by
MPG Books Ltd, Bodmin, Cornwall

Contents

List of Tables and Boxes

Tables

Boxes

Acknowledgements

We would like to extend our thanks to various members of our families who have had to tolerate us working so arduously, especially latterly, on this book.

We would like to acknowledge Miss Greta Depledge for help with typing and staff at the Royal Free Hospital for support.

Preface

Surinder Singh and Sara Madge review the total spectrum of HIV infection from diagnosis to death of those infected. They make a significant contribution towards comprehensive care by suggesting ways that a variety of health and social care providers in the primary care setting can deal with those who are infected and affected.

In the late 1990s, the diagnosis, treatment and care of those with HIV infection is very different from what it was in 1985. These authors emphasise that HIV is now a chronic rather than an acute condition. A range of health and social care providers need to be aware of the constantly changing profile of HIV. The thrust of this change comes from better diagnostic and monitoring tests alongside more effective combinations of anti-retroviral therapies. In 1985 there were less medical and social reasons for people to be diagnosed with HIV. Early diagnosis enables individuals to consider newer treatment options.

What this book does refreshingly is to take the mystique out of many aspects of HIV diagnosis and care. The authors suggest that care can be, and should be, shared between HIV specialist centres and the community services. The contents cover both practical information (living wills, guardianship, advanced directives and advice about registration with a general practitioner) as well as some of the more complex issues such as depression and psychiatric illness in the context of HIV.

This text clearly highlights the parameters between the expertise provided by HIV specialist centres and the care that can complement this in the community. The documentation of the authors' views are timely. Closer liaison between primary and secondary care with shorter hospital admissions and follow-up care in the community is needed. The authors offer more than 'lip service' to the notion of collaborative multidisciplinary care. They offer a comprehensive analysis of problems faced by people with HIV and their families and friends, as well as practical solutions which are grounded in their day-to-day practice both in hospitals and the community.

From different standpoints both authors are also well-placed to offer up-to-date information and ideas about dealing with all stages of HIV infection. The changing profile of HIV infection emphasises that specialist centres need to offer easy access to diagnosis, assessment, monitoring and treatment but that liaison with general practitioners is vital if patients are to receive optimal care for themselves and their families.

The authors emphasise how different professionals, working together, can help reduce HIV transmission and enhance the care of those patients with HIV. Health and social care professionals other than doctors may be the first to suspect HIV as a differential diagnosis and should feel comfortable enough to raise the subject. The population most at risk are young, healthy, and of child-bearing age. The authors indicate how opportunities can be taken to reduce transmission and diagnose HIV by raising the issue more routinely alongside other health issues such as smoking, drugs, contraception and travel. Assumptions should also not be made about who is at risk. Particularly relevant for those in the community is the discussion and testing for HIV with women and their partners before and during pregnancy to reduce the transmission of HIV from mother to infant. Basic information about HIV, which is presented in a straightforward, accurate and not too technical style, should be helpful to readers.

The chosen focus of primary care helps us to find more successful ways forward to reduce fears of stigma and discrimination associated with HIV by considering issues surrounding confidentiality in HIV alongside all other illnesses. Primary care is where HIV discussion must start. It is hoped that a range of health and social care professionals will be able to approach HIV more routinely and with less reluctance after reading the case histories. This text shows how this can be done. Its clearly written information presented in a clear, accessible format helps to dispel the myths surrounding the counselling, diagnosis, treatment and care of HIV infected patients and their families and loved ones.

Riva Miller
Family Therapist and AIDS Counselling Coordinator
Honorary Senior Lecturer
Royal Free Hospital NHS Trust and Royal Free School of Medicine

1 The History of HIV Infection and Transmission

Introduction

It is both prudent and necessary to ask why another book on HIV and AIDS? Surely enough has been written on the subject already? We think not and here's why. This book is aimed primarily at personnel such as social workers, care workers and care assistants. The book may well appeal to district and community nurses, including practice nurses who need to know about HIV infection and AIDS, but who do not wish to become too involved in the intricacies of these inter-related conditions. These various groups may be complemented by trainee nurses or trainee clinicians from other disciplines. We would also be interested to know if this book was used by family, friends or the loved ones of those affected by chronic HIV infection or AIDS. The one commonality is that they will be involved with people affected by, and sometimes infected with, chronic HIV infection and AIDS in the community – in other words, in people's homes.

The aim of this book is to serve several functions:

- It provides important and key information about HIV infection and AIDS.
- It provides, through various means, a uniquely community approach to the care of people with HIV infection.
- It aims to inform health care workers that the challenge about caring for people with HIV infection is one which can and, importantly, should be an ordinary and routine component of primary care services.

We would be grateful to know the extent to which these aims have or have

1

not been met.

The book is divided into three main sections. The first section, Chapters 1 to 4, is devoted to the natural history of HIV infection including details about basic immunology, pathology, epidemiology and the evolving nature of the global pandemic. Chapter 2 is specifically about prevention of HIV infection – really the only meaningful weapon so far – against HIV and AIDS. The last chapter of this section is on advancing disease, when HIV infection has resulted in significant damage to the body's immunity so that it is vulnerable to a host of infections. The second section, Chapters 5 to 8, focuses on mental health issues and HIV/AIDS medications. This section also contains two separate chapters on the primary care team and the hospital team, because these two 'teams' can play a fairly central role in the clinical care of a person with HIV infection or AIDS.

The third section, Chapters 9 to 11, form the central core of this book. Chapter 9 attempts to explore complex issues in HIV care, for example families, including children, where more than one member is infected with the virus. Other issues such as dealing with uncertainty, which seems to be an inherent part of HIV and AIDS, is also a feature. This chapter also examines change, another consistent aspect of HIV and AIDS. Chapter 10 starts off where Chapter 4 finished, contemplating what to expect if a person with HIV becomes increasingly weak or incapacitated by HIV infection or one of its many complications. The community aspects of this section are emphasised because it is the views of the authors that patient choice is enhanced by care at home, so long as it is planned and anticipated. This section is completed by Chapter 11 which clarifies and hopefully demystifies some of the practicalities surrounding the death of a loved one at home or in hospital.

At the end of the book are a list of useful addresses and contact numbers, a glossary and a comprehensive reading list. The book is completed by the index.

The beginning of the global HIV epidemic

It is tragically ironic that in 1978, at the time of the momentous 'Health for All by the Year 2000' declaration by the World Health Organisation (WHO) the global HIV and AIDS epidemic was well under way, albeit unknowingly. How were the first cluster of 'cases' detected?

In what is now almost medical folklore, the first people to be identified with HIV were in the United States in 1980, because their 'marker conditions' were very unusual. It is important to emphasise at this stage that AIDS, the Acquired Immune Deficiency Syndrome, is a collection of individual diseases which are defined by the World Health Organisation (WHO). There are unfortunately some significant differences in the definitions between the US and Europe and these will be discussed later.

What made the original marker conditions unusual, the two most common being pneumocystis carinii pneumonia (PCP) and Kaposi's sarcoma (KS), was that these were normally associated with people who were already very ill, often with underlying cancers, lymphomas or who had had organ transplant surgery, for example a kidney transplant. The one factor which linked such groups of patients was that their immune systems were not functioning as well as they could, hence the initial theory that the causative agent (not identified until three years later) had an adverse influence on the immunity of those individuals affected. It was also apparent that these earliest cases occurred in young men whose commonality was that they were gay. Thus, the link was made between a condition which associated homosexuality, or to be more accurate penetrative sexual intercourse, with a state of 'poor' immunity.

It is remarkable that in the last 15 years great and significant strides have been made in elucidating and confirming various aspects of the collection of conditions now called AIDS. Thus, following a series of unbecoming names, for example GRID – gay-related immuno-deficiency disease, the virus causing the underlying immunity problem was identified in 1983 in France and the US and called the human immuno-deficiency virus (HIV). While some minority sources continue to question whether the human immuno-deficiency virus is the actual cause of AIDS, it is becoming increasingly clear through a variety of epidemiological studies, that globally HIV is almost certainly the cause of AIDS. It is important to state that while the epidemic in the USA was growing, in other parts of the world, such as Africa, the spread of HIV has also been inexorable and relentless.

The confirmation of HIV infection (HIV-1) has been possible through retrospective testing and, apparently, through post-mortem tissues still in existence. It is widely accepted that one of the first ever confirmed cases of AIDS was in a Norwegian sailor, who was infected in the early 1960s and died in 1976 (Hooper 1997). Tragically his wife and eleven-year-old daughter also died at about the same time.

The intriguing feature about this sexually active sailor (he acquired gonorrhoea soon after his fifteenth birthday) was that he frequently sailed along the west coast of Africa where in countries like Cameroon, Côte-d'Ivoire, Gabon, HIV was later to become endemic. There have been other similar and sporadic reports from other European countries about early cases of AIDS-like syndromes, for example in Germany where a bisexual male died of possible AIDS in 1979, and in France where a child died in 1981 'following a clinical history highly suggestive of neonatal AIDS'. In 1992 the virus was isolated from the mother who, by then, had AIDS.

In the end, how the human immuno-deficiency virus (HIV) finally emerged is far from clear. Perhaps it arose in a few places at about the same time (like a 'starburst'), perhaps from its nearest 'cousin' – the simian (monkey) immuno-deficiency virus. More worryingly, the well-intentioned but flawed 'hand of medical science' may have played its part: it has been suggested that monkeys were bred, killed, then used to produce vaccines for human subjects and somewhere along this route HIV emerged (Hooper 1997). The theory is that HIV has been present for many years, however it is only since the early 1980s that somehow it has become more aggressive and potent. The reasons for this adverse change remains unknown though clearly environmental, local and geo-demographic factors may all play a part.

Box 1.1   Important landmarks in HIV/AIDS history

1980: First cases identified in the US
1983: Virus isolated for first time simultaneously in the US and France
1987: First anti-retroviral medication launched by Wellcome
1990: Global pandemic worsening but impact is different on First and Third World countries
1996: New hope at the Vancouver AIDS Conference: can HIV be eliminated?

What exactly is HIV?

The human immuno-deficiency virus is first and foremost a virus whose central core structure is composed of ribonucleic acid (RNA). (Most viruses, and there are many different types, are composed of deoxyribonucleic acid – DNA.) Ultimately it is this genetic material which determines the qualities of the virus (see Chapter 3). Other types of virus cause other diseases, many of which are mild but irritating (like the common cold or flu), while others, for example, the cold sore (herpes simplex type 1) are more troublesome and can be persistent. Another type of herpes, called herpes simplex type 2 is associated with genital ulcers which are intermittent, can be very nasty and are invariably sexually transmitted (see Chapter 3).

Some viruses, for example polio, measles or rubella, can be entirely prevented though a series of vaccinations; these last examples form part of the UK national immunisation programme for children and are vital in ensuring conditions such as rubella are relatively rare. Nevertheless all these are infections caused by viruses. In what has been called the World Health Organisation's greatest single feat, smallpox – another viral infection – was eradicated in the late 1980s. It is a long-term hope that the same can happen to HIV infection.

The structure of the human immuno-deficiency virus (HIV) has a number of features which make it unique. First, the virus' RNA – the chromosomal building blocks of the virus – is surrounded by a protein core with an overlying protein-sugar 'coat'. The configuration of the 'coat' allows HIV to attach itself to human cells during the infective process. More specifically it attaches itself to certain cell types within the human immune system – the T4 lymphocytes, sometimes called CD4 cells. These same cells are sometimes called 'helper' or 'inducer' CD4 cells; all these terms are synonymous. In addition HIV also infects other 'immune-related' cells in the body, for example macrophages which are cells that 'gobble up' bacterial and viral debris. These cells play an absolutely vital role in orchestrating the body's response to infections from viruses, or other 'germs' such as bacteria which are almost ubiquitous in our ordinary environments. Once these cells are infected, HIV can remain dormant for many months or years in a process which is, as yet, incompletely understood.

What happens next is the key to why HIV is so difficult to eradicate and why, fundamentally it causes so much damage. This damage occurs after a prolonged period, though the exact time period is largely undetermined in individual patients. The virus's chromosomal material, composed of the RNA now converts this into DNA using its own enzyme 'reverse transcriptase'. After a period of time the contaminated material is turned into many other copies of the immuno-deficiency virus though these remain well hidden within the central core structure (genome) of the host cell. The virus replicates quite rapidly, but often unsuccessfully. During this time it is almost as if there is a status quo established between the virus and the host.

However, because viral activity continues over a sustained period, millions of viruses are ultimately produced. While initially the body is able to replace the important CD4 cells, this cannot occur indefinitely. Eventually, the CD4 cells cannot maintain their numbers in the face of persistent and continuing HIV replication and their numbers start to decline.

As the virus replicates itself almost endlessly, so many CD4 cells are lost that the body cannot replace them. The immune system becomes increasingly depressed and compromised and thus becomes vulnerable to infections and tumours which are the hallmark of advanced HIV disease. Minor, and then major, health problems start to manifest themselves. It is not known what factors influence the length of the asymptomatic, 'dormant period' – suffice it to say that many of these as yet remain unknown or subject to much debate and controversy within the scientific community.

This information should therefore help you to understand why HIV is so difficult to eradicate; it should also explain that the period from initial infection to the development of serious illness can be very long, in some cases well over 15 years. Once again, these details remain unknown despite the welter of research since HIV first appeared. The production of a vaccination remains a major challenge, very simply because the exact structure of HIV's RNA is ever-changing and 'mutating', due to a variety of reasons. In contrast, the reason there is a highly effective vaccine for rubella is that the composition of rubella virus is relatively stable and thus a single vaccine provides ample protection. This is not the case with HIV.

Finally, scientists believe that HIV is not one entity which is the same the world over. Epidemiological evidence strongly suggests that various sub-types of HIV exist, each responsible for its own mini-epidemic, though clearly there is crossover of infection from one region of the world to another. Moreover, it is these sub-types which may be responsible for the variation in transmission patterns. So far just less than ten types (labelled A to I) have been identified. For example, sub-types A, C and D predominate in Africa where the vast majority of infections occur heterosexually. In Europe and North America it is sub-type B which is more prevalent, while in India sub-type C is more common. In Thailand it is thought that two epidemics have occurred, the first due to sub-type B has been spread through injecting drug users, while sub-type E has infected individuals heterosexually. These differences reflect subtle differences in the anatomical features of the HIV particles and may influence how each virus attaches itself to the cells of the genitalia (see Chapter 3).

How is HIV infection transmitted?

It has been known for a long time that HIV can only be transmitted through well-recognised ways, the most common being through sexual intercourse. Early in the epidemic, gay men appeared to be those most affected by this new condition – however, *it is not being gay that is the causal factor*. Very simply, any individual having penetrative vaginal or anal sex – quite a common occurrence when considering this in a global context – can be at risk of acquiring HIV infection. It is extremely important to remember that world-wide the most common mode of transmission is through heterosexual sexual intercourse.

The central feature of transmission is that there is an exchange of body fluids, and in the context of a person infected with HIV, every body fluid has been found to contain the virus: blood, saliva, semen, vaginal fluid, sweat and tears. This fact does not necessarily mean that all these 'fluids' transmit the virus with the same propensity.

World-wide the most important modes of transmission are:

Box 1.2   Known routes of HIV transmission

Penetrative sexual intercourse
* Women who have sex with men, men who have sex with women (heterosexual)
* Men who have sex with men (gay, homosexual)
* Individuals who have sex with women and men (bisexual)
* Oral sex

Inoculation of blood
* Inoculation of infected blood and blood products
* Needle-sharing among injecting drug-users
* Injections with unsterile needles
* Needle-stick injuries

Perinatal
* Inter-uterine transmission from mother to foetus
* Peripartum i.e. through breast-feeding

Box 1.3   Routes *not* shown to be involved with HIV transmission

* Close personal contacts, including using eating and drinking utensils
* Ordinary social kissing
* Household contacts, including sharing towels and toilets
* Using swimming pools and jacuzzis
* Professional contact with health care workers including doctors and dentists
* Insect bites

Infection control

It is prudent at this stage to discuss the obvious ways of minimising any chance of acquiring HIV infection through accidents or injuries. Infections occurring in health care workers receive more than their fair share of publicity, much of it negative and often salacious; however, the chances of acquiring infection through this route is very small. Where health care workers have become infected it is usually because of other 'activities', such as sexual intercourse. Where an infection has occurred occupationally it is usually because workers have not taken ordinary precautions, which ought to be carried out on all patients, whether identified as HIV-positive or (and much more likely) whose HIV status is unknown. These precautions are also important for other infections, for example hepatitis B, which is often also prevalent in certain groups of people with HIV infection, for example gay men, people with haemophilia and injecting drug-users (see Chapter 2).

One of the most effective barriers against infection of any type for the human body is the skin, indeed it is one of the functions of this organ. Thus one important strategy to ensure your protection against HIV is to maximise this natural barrier and minimise preventable and unforeseen breaches in the skin.

Washing hands and using gloves

Washing hands is an absolute must for all health care workers and should never be overlooked; while so far the emphasis has been on the protection of the health worker, it is important to realise that potentially the health care worker poses more of a risk to the patient than the reverse. This is especially so if you are seeing a number of patients during the same session, for example, during home visits. Where possible it is good practice to wash hands with soap and hot water before and after seeing patients and especially after any 'procedure'. In addition – and this is irrespective of HIV infection – it is also good practice to wash hands before the preparation and eating of food.

Wearing gloves is important where handling body fluids, whatever the source of the body fluid. If the contact person has breaches in the skin, for example due to a cut, then a simple precaution is to use a plaster covering. If the skin is affected in other ways, for example due to eczema or psoriasis, it is sensible that this work should be avoided. A common-sense perspective is necessary here – if the care worker has a minute, barely visible crack in the skin, then so long as gloves are worn, the overall risk will be negligible.

Cleaning up body excretions usually necessitates a two-stage process: first the excretions are removed using hot soapy water (gloves are mandatory in this instance), and second, the area is disinfected using 10 per cent hypochlorite solution (one part household bleach to ten parts of hot water). Remember not to use bleach directly on skin since this will burn. And also remember bleach on carpets, furnishings and clothes will invariably ruin them! Where bleach is used, ensure good ventilation in order that the powerful fumes can escape without causing any harm to people in the vicinity.

Commodes and bedpans will need regular cleaning, especially where there is incontinence or problems with diarrhoea and soiling. In these circumstances, gloves and disposable gowns can be used in order to ensure protection and prevent damage to clothes. Where clothes have been soiled, a 'hot wash' in a washing machine, sometimes complemented with bleach, will be all that is necessary.

Needles and sharps

Needles and sharps probably represent the major risk for health professionals. However, with a few basic guidelines, these can be minimised to the point where overall risk is negligible:

1. Take your time.
2. Do not re-sheath needles.
3. Needles and other sharps ought to be placed immediately in a 'sharps bin', a specially designed puncture-resistant bin which can be portable.

Accidents occur when health professionals become complacent and flout the obvious precautions, or when they are in a hurry, perhaps for good reason such as the 'emergency situation'. A combination of factors can prove to be dangerous. It is important that the 'sharps bin' should not be over-filled since this increases the chances of a needle-stick injury.

This sub-section is merely a summary and is discussed in detail in Chapter 2 under 'Nosocomial infection'.

A global perspective

Globally, and it certainly is a global pandemic, the manifestations of HIV, including AIDS, pose a direct challenge to politicians, health care workers, employees, local communities and families. It is estimated that by the year 2000, approximately thirty to forty million people will be infected with HIV, and the largest proportions will be in the so-called developing countries. In the last three years prior to the new millennium, there are an estimated eight-and-a-half million people with AIDS, though exact numbers are difficult to obtain because of under-reporting, the inevitable delays in reporting and, crucially, under-recognition (UNAIDS 1996). Africa, South America and, increasingly, South-east Asia bear the brunt of the evolving epidemic.

According to UNAIDS estimates, there have been over three million new cases of HIV infection during 1996 alone, working out at 8,500 per day, 1,000 of whom are children. In the same year, HIV/AIDS-associated illnesses caused the death of an estimated one and a half million people, including 350,000 children. Overall in a global context 1 in a 100 people are HIV-positive. The male to female ratio is about two to one, but this is beginning to equalise rapidly.

Mode of transmission

In Europe and North America, much is made of the high prevalence rates in gay and bisexual individuals and who, as previously stated, were the groups initially affected. Sexual transmission was the prime transmission mode in these areas. Similarly, world-wide about eighty per cent of all infections occur through penetrative sexual intercourse. However, globally seventy per cent of these infections occur heterosexually; male–male intercourse (gay, homosexual) account for a further five to ten per cent of all cases. In other words, there is a 'heterosexual' to 'homosexual' ratio of seven to one. In Europe and the US, these proportions differ markedly: in the UK, approximately seventy per cent of all known cases of AIDS occur in people who are gay or bisexual, in stark contrast to the pattern of world-wide statistics of those infected (UNAIDS 1996). It is increasingly recognised that the presence of other more traditional sexually-transmitted infections, for example gonorrhoea or syphilis, paves the way for HIV infection.

Approximately fifteen per cent of all infants born to women with HIV infection themselves become infected with the virus, either before, during or after birth (through breast-feeding). In the West, breast-feeding is not recommended for babies born to infected women. Unfortunately, in developing countries, the situation is more complex and since the mortality of a young child suffering with gastroenteritis is exceedingly high this decision is a difficult one. In fact, most observers agree that breast-feeding in these circumstances is beneficial despite the risk of transmitting HIV infection.

People who share equipment when injecting drugs also incur a major risk for the simple reason that 'the equipment' is often contaminated. World-wide this group accounts for about ten per cent of all infections, though in southern Europe this represents the main route of transmission resulting in very high rates amongst injecting drug-users. Transfusions of HIV-infected blood or products account for between three and five per cent of all infections. A rational policy of using voluntary blood donors and, in many countries, of blood-screening now means that this mode of transmission should continue to decrease with time. It is salutary to note that some countries do not have such screening procedures in place because of resource implications.

HIV-2

So far HIV infection has been discussed as if it is a single infective agent. Unfortunately this is not the case and a another type of HIV, named HIV-2 (the original is sometimes called HIV-1) has a different genetic composition. HIV-2 was originally identified from West Africa though has now been found in other places such as Asia and Latin America. It is certainly marginal in comparison with HIV-1 as far as global figures are concerned. In addition, it appears to be transmitted less easily than HIV-1 and the clinical course is slower and perhaps more indolent (UNAIDS 1996). Treatment for HIV-2 is the same as for HIV-1 though, as stated, this is rare in the UK.

The evolving epidemic

The dynamic of the problem of HIV, as has been the case since it appeared in the early 1980s, is that it is evolving and perhaps, the worst is yet to come (Mann 1992). In the developed world where HIV has appeared in large numbers, the infection continues to spread, especially in the larger conurbations such as New York, San Francisco and other cities. While the overall number of new infections has decreased in such communities, largely due to significantly successful behaviour-changing campaigns over the last ten years, a new generation of gay and bisexual men appear to be disregarding this problem to their cost. The result is that in more recent studies younger men, aged between 17 and 22 years, are now becoming infected.

In some countries, there has been a meteoric rise in numbers in the last few years, perhaps in places which did not record their first cases until the mid 1990s. Central and eastern European countries illustrate this phenomena quite poignantly, though it is important to state the factors for this are multiple, complex and invariably inter-related (economic survival, prostitution, injected opiates and a 'sexual revolution'). In the Ukraine, HIV prevalence amongst a group of drug users rose dramatically from just under two per cent to nearly 60 per cent within the same year. In Russia the rapid rise in numbers is replicated through various regions and cities, for example, in Kaliningrad the numbers of people infected rose 18-fold since the beginning of 1996, again due to a growing number of people sharing contaminated injection equipment. Even more worrying, in the newer independent republics sexually-transmitted disease (STD) rates have doubled and sometimes quadrupled in the last three years. While monitoring these other 'marker' infections has its problems, the implications for HIV infection are plain for all to see.

The real burden is being felt in those African countries which some have regarded as the original epicentre of the pandemic. Approximately 14 million people with HIV infection or AIDS live in African countries, representing over 60 per cent of the total world figure. In countries such as Kenya, Uganda, Zambia and Zimbabwe, ten per cent of women attending antenatal clinics are infected with HIV; this number rises to 40 per cent in some surveillance sites. Most of Africa is involved and southern African countries including South Africa have alarmingly high rates of infection. Continuing demographic changes, such as the move from rural to urban areas and the major disruption experienced by countries with highest prevalence rates, such as Zaire and Rwanda, means that the course of the HIV and AIDS epidemic will be unpredictably severe.

The highest rates of HIV infection are now in South-East Asia; as a result, the number of HIV cases here will overtake the number occurring in the African sub-continent before long. Countries such as Thailand, India and Burma point to a volatility of the epidemic which could only be estimated in 'worst-case scenarios' a few years ago. In Bombay the prevalence rates of sex workers with HIV is 50 per cent in one study, while it is 36 per cent in people attending STD clinics. Two-and-a-half per cent of all women attending antenatal clinics are HIV-positive. The danger is that, as in Africa, the epidemic will spread to rural areas. A study has shown that five to ten per cent of truck drivers in certain Indian areas have chronic HIV infection. As in Africa, since people feel healthy and look healthy, very few of these highly mobile workers are identified. They act – though clearly unwittingly – as highly efficient transmitters of HIV infection along the byroads and routes of the large highways. The true level of this burden of infection will not be known for some time yet.

The countries reporting the largest numbers of HIV-infected individuals in Europe include France, Spain, Italy and Switzerland. A microcosm of the great variability which has just been described can be seen in the UK.

Using unlinked anonymous testing figures and other data, it is possible to estimate the total number of prevalent infections, that is those people who are alive with HIV infection. 'Unlinked' testing means that there is no way of being able to identify a particular patient from this type of testing, even if it was decided that a 'positive result' ought to be identified as an individual. 'Anonymous' testing means that neither doctors/nurses nor patients know that the test is being done, and because it is unlinked consent is not an issue. Testing is carried out in a variety of settings, for example, in out-patient departments, GP surgeries, clinics for injecting drug-users and antenatal clinics. The purpose of doing these tests is to estimate from a wide variety of sources the total number of people with HIV infection in a given population. Unlinked, anonymous testing is much more of an epidemiological tool, in other words, it is used for the tracking of an epidemic, in this case HIV infection, over a period of time. The main limitation of this testing is that there is no way to translate back to each individual person.

In terms of comparison with Europe and beyond, it is clear from such data that the UK has a low population prevalence of HIV. The countries with the highest working estimates of HIV seroprevalence are Spain (where it approaches 0.6 per cent of the population), Switzerland (less than 0.3 per cent), Italy, France, Belgium and Austria. Yugoslavia, Greece, Ireland, Malta, Germany, Luxembourg, Iceland, Denmark and Portugal all have a higher estimated prevalence than the United Kingdom (DOH 1996).

Thus, while in England and Wales the figures are closely allied to those in the US, in other words, the majority of people known to have HIV and AIDS are gay or bisexual, the profile in Scotland is markedly different again. Here, because of an almost unique set of circumstances in the late 1970s and early 1980s, the commonest cause of HIV transmission was through sharing needles. As a result, the number of women infected with HIV is more than double that of the UK as a whole. In addition, male to female and female to male transmission has contributed to the escalating figures in Scotland. Almost a quarter of the total number of people with HIV infection (as opposed to AIDS) are women. The indications are that by the new century almost a quarter of those developing AIDS will be women (Bury 1992).

In England the largest number of people with HIV infection and AIDS are confined to those in the biggest conurbations, the most notable being London. It is still the case that two out of every three cases of AIDS are in people who reside in the two Thames Regions (CDR 1997). A number of surveys and research projects over the past few years have revealed that almost 90 per cent of general practitioners have seen and treated people with AIDS in the period leading up to the survey (Hoolaghan 1992). There are nearly 30,000 individuals with HIV infection in the UK, almost 14,000 of whom have developed AIDS. Almost 10,000 people have died with AIDS since the early 1980s.

Risk groups or risk activities?

It was common, perhaps all too common, especially at the beginning of the epidemic, to discuss 'risk groups', as if it was the belonging to a group that conferred upon an individual a higher risk of acquiring HIV infection or AIDS. It is much more sensible and rational to discuss this in the context of 'risk activities', since, as is mentioned earlier, it is these which are important and not the risk-group stereotypes.

Engaging in penetrative, unprotected sex with a man or a woman confers risk. Early advertising campaigns stressed the need to be vigilant, that having sex with a new partner, effectively meant having sex with all his or her other partners. There is a certain sense to this, though the presentation of health messages like this does not appeal to everyone. Of course, the answer to the question 'How can I remain completely safe from infection?' is to not have penetrative, unprotected sexual intercourse. However, for the majority of people this seems rather extreme and unnecessarily unpleasant. There is always safe(r) sex.

Safe sex

Totally safe sex probably does not exist. 'Safer sex' is a better term for the concepts described in this section. An important component of this term, which seems to be the prime ingredient of any health promotion, is that it is absolutely impossible to identify from appearance alone if a person is infected with HIV. Thus, as is stated above, there is something to be said for the argument that having sex with someone who is unfamiliar is akin to having sex with their partners before them, be they male or female. Common sense would dictate that if a man has had sex with another man, or has injected drugs, or has spent time in countries where HIV infection is more prevalent, the chance of that person having this infection is going to be higher. If none of these factors are present then there is less risk. Of course, if it is impossible to 'assess' the person (whatever this means) it may be easier and pragmatic to assume that HIV is amongst one of many sexually transmitted diseases which can be prevented by practising safe(r) sex.

What therefore is safer sex? There are lists of what is and what is not safer sex; for example low-risk activities clearly will not involve penetration; these activities include kissing, massage, partner masturbation, oral sex and using sex toys. Once again, with this highly theoretical list, oral sex shall be regarded as *low* risk, not *no*-risk, though again the chances of HIV transmission are remarkably low. The same applies to the use of sex toys.

The latex, male condom is a common protection, used world-wide against many sexually transmitted diseases. However, condoms belong in the safer-sex category since they can burst, split or even fall off; however the main reason for failure is that they are not used properly. There are now male and female condoms; the latter are being marketed in many countries and are based upon the same principle as male condoms: they act as a barrier to sperm and also 'infections'. Though it is potentially more woman-focused, some women find using the female condom (the femidom) problematic; certainly it is better than no protection at all (see Chapter 2 for further details).

In either case both the contraceptive and HIV protective properties of such condoms are greatly enhanced if used in conjunction with a spermicide, a chemical compound which kills off sperm, is potentially toxic to HIV, and is usually used to enhance the effectiveness of the condoms or the diaphragm to prevent pregnancy. Most condoms, though not all, are treated with spermicide, hence supplying another level of protection, though the extent of this extra protection will always be difficult to gauge.

Is a cure for HIV/AIDS on the horizon?

There has been much speculation that a cure for HIV infection is on the horizon; unfortunately, this is probably not true, not though there is much room for a guarded optimism which was not the case even three years ago.

There has been a key breakthrough in how HIV can be treated with a major announcement at the Vancouver World AIDS Conference in the summer of 1996. This mainly centred on the finding that, using several anti-viral compounds in some patients (traditionally called 'combination therapies'), the activity of HIV infection could be curtailed to *almost* nothing. Of course, this raises many questions: what types of medications are being used? How long should treatments be used? How available are they and are there long-term side-effects? Some of these points will be discussed in later chapters.

In addition, HIV monitoring in an HIV-positive person has become more sophisticated: actual CD4 counts can now be combined with new measurements of 'viral load', which altogether raises the accuracy and precision with which monitoring can take place on an individual patient basis (see Chapters 2 and 3).

Finally, in the area of antenatal care, evidence suggests that the rate of perinatal transmission can be vastly reduced using several well-known and none-too-aggressive measures. For example, the rate of transmission to the foetus can be cut by two-thirds if the woman is already on Zidovudine (the first anti-retroviral treatment and sometimes called AZT), if the delivery is through a Caesarian section and if breast-feeding is disallowed. It goes without saying that, for the woman with HIV infection, these decisions must be based on a frank and open discussion between clinician – usually a doctor – and patient, not imposed or forced upon her. It is prudent to mention that for the majority of the world's population of people with HIV infection, these treatments and precautions remain nothing but empty theory. The consistent lack of resources for some countries means that such therapies, which cost the equivalent of thousands of pounds per patient per year, are simply not available for the majority of people (Beiser 1997, Cohn 1997). Even in the UK, there is discussion that funding of these therapies will only happen if savings are found in other clinical areas, for example, community HIV services (Bury 1997, personal communication).

References

Beiser, C. (1997) 'HIV infection-2', *British Medical Journal*, 314: 579–583.

Bury, J. (1992), 'Women and the AIDS epidemic: some medical facts and figures' in Bury, Judy, Morrison, Val and McLachlan, Sheena (eds), *Working with women and AIDS*, London: Tavistock/Routledge.

Cohn, J.A. (1997) 'HIV infection-1', *British Medical Journal*, 314: 487–491.

CDR (Communicable Disease Report) (1997) 'The epidemiology of HIV infection and AIDS', *CDR*, Vol. 7 (review no. 9), August.

Department of Health Report (1996) 'Unlinked Anonymous HIV Prevalence Monitoring Programme, England and Wales', London: Department of Health.

Hoolaghan, Tony (1992), 'Health Promotion in General Practice Project', London: Hampstead Health Promotion Project.

Hooper, E. (1997) 'Sailors & starbursts, and the arrival of HIV', *British Medical Journal*, 315: 1689–91.

Mann, Jonathan (1992) 'AIDS in the 1990s: A Global analysis', Malcom Morris Memorial Lecture, *Journal of the Royal Society of Health*, 112 (3), June.

UNAIDS (1996) *The right to care*, Bulletin from the Joint United Nations Programme on HIV/AIDS, Geneva: UNAIDS.

2   HIV Prevention

HIV can be passed on in several ways, most commonly through unprotected penetrative sex, as well as through shared needles and syringe use. In the past in the United Kingdom, HIV was transmitted through blood and blood products. HIV can also be transmitted nosocomially: that is through the workplace from patient to health worker or vice versa. Finally HIV can be transmitted from mother to child. This is called vertical transmission and will be discussed later in this chapter.

Sexual transmission of HIV

HIV is most commonly passed on through heterosexual sex, that is, vaginal sex between a man and a woman. HIV is transmitted through sex via body fluids: semen in men and vaginal fluid in women.

Condom use

When a man or a woman who has HIV has unprotected vaginal sex with someone else there are several important factors that determine whether or not the virus is passed on. The most effective way to reduce the rate of HIV transmission (apart from having non-penetrative sex) is to use a condom.

Using a condom will dramatically reduce the chances of HIV being passed on because it acts as a barrier between the mixing of body fluids that occurs during unprotected sex. Most condoms also contain spermicides which have been shown to kill HIV. Sex with a condom is very safe; however, it is well-known that condom use does not fully protect someone from HIV (as shown by the number of women who become pregnant while using condoms as a form of contraception). The most common reason for 'condom failure' is that the condom can split or burst. Condoms are often *used incorrectly*, making them more likely to tear. For example, people need to be aware that, when using condoms with a teat at the end, the teat *must* be held while putting on the condom; otherwise, air may get into it making it more likely to split. In addition, some men only put on condoms just before ejaculation. This is risky because some semen is produced before ejaculation and in this way HIV may be transmitted in the pre-ejaculate.

Condoms also have *different thicknesses*. Those that are thinner are more likely to split. Condoms that are of a sufficiently high standard are marked with a British 'kitemark'. People often receive conflicting advice about the various types of condoms and how they should be used. If this is the case, sources of guidance include the general practitioner (GP), family planning clinic and the local genito-urinary clinic. Health advisers who usually work in the genito-urinary clinics are specially trained sexual health counsellors and a reliable source of help.

In recent years a female condom (the femidom) has been developed. This can also protect against HIV and other sexually transmitted diseases. They can be bought in chemists, but they are a little more complicated to use as they need to fit over the cervix (the neck of the womb). Many people would need advice about how this ought to be used; again good sources of advice include the family doctor, the practice nurse or family planning nurses.

The cap or diaphragm is a form of contraceptive which prevents pregnancy by forming a barrier between the cervix and the penis. It does not offer full protection against HIV for women as only the cervix is covered. The vaginal walls are not protected from the mixing of body fluids. The cap should always be used with a spermicide.

Some women choose to use condoms as their only form of contraception. However, given the risk of condoms bursting, women may choose to use the oral contraceptive pill as well so that they are doubly protected from becoming pregnant. The method whereby women use both the oral contraceptive pill and the condom to protect against pregnancy and sexually transmitted diseases was pioneered in Holland and has been described as the 'double-Dutch' method of contraception (not a very edifying name!).

If condom breakage occurs, pregnancy can also be avoided by using the 'morning-after' pill which is easily prescribed by GPs or family planning centres. It is highly effective up to 72 hours after a condom failure, or unprotected intercourse. Two pills are given at the time the woman presents to the doctor and then two further pills are given twelve hours later. The 'morning-after' pill does not guarantee that pregnancy will not occur but it reduces the risk substantially. The main side effect is nausea. Sometimes women are given anti-nausea pills to take at the same time, or are given advice that should they vomit after taking the morning-after pill they should return to the doctors for further assessment. If a woman presents between three and five days after condom failure then it is possible for an intra-uterine device (IUCD or coil) to be fitted as a short-term measure to reduce the risk of pregnancy. Neither of these measures are 'fail-safe', however they reduce the risk of pregnancy in such circumstances.

Sexually transmitted diseases (STDs)

HIV is more likely to be transmitted if a person has a co-existing sexually transmitted disease (STD), particularly if this takes the form of an ulcer, that is, a broken skin surface through which HIV can be transmitted. It also appears that people with HIV, who also have other sexually transmitted diseases, may 'concentrate' HIV in their body fluids making them more likely to transmit the virus. In Africa strict control of STDs has helped to reduce the spread of HIV in some communities (Grosskurth et al. 1995). In the United Kingdom too, encouraging people to have regular check-ups for STDs may have also reduced the spread of HIV.

People with HIV are usually offered regular screening for STDs in their hospital clinics. Genito-urinary (GU) clinics will see anyone who is concerned about HIV or other sexually transmitted diseases. It is not necessary to be referred by a general practitioner (although they can do). Most GPs are not able to do all the specialist investigations that a GU clinic can perform. Moreover, genito-urinary clinics can provide some results of tests, and therefore treatment, on the day of testing.

It is important to screen for STDs as many of these cause no obvious symptoms and yet can be quite serious, causing many problems later on if not treated. For example, chlamydia, an infection which is very easily treated, causes infertility in women if persistent or left untreated for long periods. It is also infamous for manifesting little or no symptoms in male partners.

Women are more likely than men to acquire HIV: the vaginal lining and cervix has a larger surface area that is more likely to be traumatised during sex. In comparison, men have a relatively small area, around the opening to the penis (urethra), which is traumatised during intercourse. In addition, HIV is more likely to be transmitted if sex is particularly traumatic or if there is blood present, for example, if the woman is menstruating.

Viral load

People with HIV have different quantities of the virus in their blood and other body fluids (see Chapter 3). It is thought that people with a high viral load, in other words a large amount of virus in their blood, are more likely to pass the virus on to others. It is not clear if people with a low level of virus in their blood necessarily have a low level of virus in the semen or vaginal fluids. Certainly even if someone has even a very low level of virus in their blood, they should still protect themselves and others by practising safer sex.

Genetic factors

Scientists also think that there are some people who are more genetically susceptible to HIV compared with others. A small proportion of people appear to have a gene that significantly reduces their chances of becoming HIV-positive. The proportion of people with this gene varies in different communities and appears to be relatively rare in Africa. The presence of this gene however may explain why a very small number of women who work as prostitutes in Kenya – one of the highest HIV-prevalence areas in the world – appear not to have become infected with HIV. The test for the HIV-resistant gene is not readily available and obviously should not be used as a reason not to take the usual precautions against HIV infection.

Research into the genetic factors involved in HIV transmission continues. It seems that the number of people who are genetically 'protected' is very small; it is also highly unlikely that this 'protection' will ever be total. Even in the unlikely event that a certain genetic make-up was found to be protective against HIV, it would not protect against other sexually transmitted infections such as hepatitis B, hepatitis C, chlamydia and other such infections.

There are other factors that may well be involved as to why some people will acquire HIV more easily that others. Experience has shown a great variety in HIV transmissibility; some people are extremely unlucky and have acquired HIV infection following sex on one occasion only, when perhaps a condom has split. Others may have unprotected sex on many occasions with an HIV-positive partner and not become HIV-positive.

Anal sex

In the gay male community, HIV is passed on largely through unprotected anal sex. However, it is important to remember that both men *and* women practise anal sex. Doctors, particularly those working in sexually-transmitted disease clinics, often need to discuss this with their patients. If two men are having unprotected anal sex, the risk of passing HIV on is much greater for the passive partner (in other words the partner who is being penetrated, receiving or 'being screwed'). This is because there is a much greater risk of trauma, and again a larger surface area, through which HIV can be transmitted to the passive partner.

Once again, the best form of protection is through condoms. Anal sex is often more traumatic as there is less natural lubrication in the anus. It is recommended that a water-based lubricant is always used when having anal sex, for example, KY jelly. Oil-based lubricants such as Vaseline are not recommended as these can cause the condom to weaken. Condoms that are recommended for anal sex are thicker and hence are stronger than those recommended for vaginal sex.

Again, condoms may break during anal sex and good condom technique is essential to ensure maximum protection. Health advisers in STD clinics can advise on the best condoms to use for anal sex and where to get them. Again it is a good idea for any man or woman who practises anal sex to go for screening for HIV and other STDs to access correct treatment and avoid complications from sexually transmitted diseases.

Oral sex

In the past it was thought that oral sex was entirely safe with respect to HIV transmission. Oral sex has now been re-categorised as 'safer sex', meaning the risk is small, but not negligible. As discussed later in Chapter 3, one common area where people with HIV infection may have symptoms is in the mouth. It is thought that if someone has gum disease, or mouth ulcers that this could be a route for transmission of HIV.

Nowadays there are many different flavours, as well as different strengths and sizes of condoms. Flavoured condoms are designed specifically for oral sex. Oral sex with a non-flavoured condom is possible though the taste of the spermicide, which is always on the outside, is not pleasant. Hence, flavoured (and sometimes coloured) condoms have been designed to encourage people to continue to use condoms for oral sex.

Again, in the context of oral sex, using condoms not only protects people from HIV but also from other sexually transmitted diseases. Many people do not realise that although unprotected oral sex is much safer than anal or vaginal sex for HIV it is not necessarily as safe for other sexually transmitted diseases. Infections which can be passed on through oral sex include herpes, gonorrhoea and syphilis.

Once people have the correct information concerning HIV transmission, what they decide to do about using condoms is very much up to them and their partner(s). Some people are so concerned about catching HIV that they do not have penetrative sex with anyone. Some people are less concerned and may decide that the small risk of HIV transmission through unprotected oral sex is acceptable for them. Others may be prepared to take more risks.

It is always difficult to decide, that if a person is continuing to expose themselves to the risk of HIV infection or other sexually transmitted diseases, what more should a health care worker do? Should the clinician or adviser continue to cajole and attempt to persuade someone, or merely accept this type of behaviour? What is important is that safer sex information is presented in an individualised user-friendly way in order to try and help a person understand that their behaviour is putting themselves and others at risk of many infections, not just HIV. It may well be unreasonable to expect anything beyond this.

Drug use

HIV is found in the blood, therefore any way in which two people mix their blood will increase the chances that HIV will be transmitted. Before we knew about the existence of HIV it was very common for people who injected drugs to share needles, syringes and other 'equipment'. After injecting themselves with a drug they might pass on the needle and syringe, which invariably would have traces of blood still inside it from the previous user. In this way a very large number of people could become infected very quickly. This is how HIV became especially common in parts of Europe, such as Spain, Italy, Switzerland and France. Once there were a number of people with HIV infected by drug use, the virus was then passed on through sex to others. In the 1980s HIV was common amongst injecting drug users in the UK, mainly in large cities, and especially in Edinburgh.

Having identified that HIV was passed on through sharing needles and syringes, several drug agencies and workers in the UK were quick to establish needle and syringe exchanges. These are now very common in most large cities in the UK where drug use is most common. By encouraging people not to re-use, but to exchange old needles and syringes for new, sterile ones, HIV has become much less common amongst people who inject drugs. Some people, however, may still find it hard to gain access to clean needles and syringes. They might live in an area where there is less drug use and services for drug users, or may be in prison.

It seems certain that drug use continues in prisons in an ever-increasing trend; sharing of needles and equipment is necessary as there is no easy access to new sterile equipment. There has been much debate as to whether needle exchanges should be established within prisons as there is evidence that HIV transmission increases in prisons (Gore et al. 1995, Gill et al. 1995).

Drug workers have also encouraged people who were injecting drug users to use their drugs in different ways other than injection, for example by smoking. This is safer, not only in terms of HIV transmission, but also other blood-borne viruses such as hepatitis B and C which can be passed on through injecting drug use. There is now a vaccination for hepatitis B which all drug users or partners of drug users should be encouraged to have in order to protect themselves. There is no vaccination to hepatitis C. While there is less known about hepatitis C, it seems that it is a more resilient virus than HIV and most people who have injected drugs for some time are infected with hepatitis C. The standard precautions which will eliminate HIV may not kill hepatitis C virus and this is also a particular area of concern for people who work with drug users.

Needle exchanges have greatly reduced the potential spread of HIV in the community. However it is important to remember that for some people in the UK, such as prisoners and for most people who inject drugs in less advantaged countries, needle exchanges are not available and are relatively costly to establish. Hence, in these situations when people will reuse needles and syringes, it is important that they are encouraged to clean equipment between use and to share it as little as possible.

In these latter circumstances, the advice is to clean needles and syringes with *cold* water twice, cleaning in between using a detergent. The reason that hot water is not recommended is that this encourages blood to congeal and some viruses, particularly hepatitis C, may be able to survive in the congealed blood. If cold water is used this is less likely to occur.

Blood products

Some people in the United Kingdom were infected with HIV through blood and blood products. This was particularly true of haemophiliacs who need a blood product (Factor 8) to help their blood clot. Many haemophiliacs have acquired HIV through blood products used before screening for HIV was standard procedure. Many are also positive for hepatitis B and hepatitis C for the same reasons.

In the UK, blood has been screened for HIV since 1985. Latterly, blood products are also heat-treated to further protect against HIV and other viruses. Nevertheless in some instances 'whole' blood is needed which needs to be fresh and therefore cannot be heat-treated.

All blood is screened for HIV by performing an HIV test shortly after blood is donated. If the HIV test and other tests performed are all negative then it is used for blood donation. There is, however, a tiny risk of acquiring HIV from a blood transfusion, because of the 'window period', which is seen in a person who is sero-converting to HIV-positive (see Chapter 3). This refers to the period of time it takes for the body to produce the antibodies in response to HIV. These antibodies are used to determine if someone is HIV-positive. It can take the body up to three months to produce enough of these antibodies to register on the HIV test. This means that an individual who donated blood, and was within this three-month window period, could theoretically escape detection. In reality this risk is much further reduced by using the constant pool of regular blood donors who are at 'low risk' for HIV. In 1997 in the UK, three people were infected with HIV from a blood donor who was in this window period. In the future other tests which can pick up HIV earlier may be used.

In many areas in the UK when people go to offer their blood for donation they are given a questionnaire prior to blood donation. This questionnaire asks them to exclude themselves if they are in a 'high-risk' group such as a gay man, injecting drug user or a person who comes from a part of the world where HIV is especially common or someone who has travelled in such an area within the last three months. Only a very small number of people who donate blood are subsequently found to be HIV-positive. They are informed by a letter asking them to return in person to the blood transfusion centre, and given the HIV-positive result in person by experienced doctors and counsellors. They are then offered medical follow-up in the usual way.

Thus, by excluding people who are potentially high risk for HIV and by using the same low-risk donors as well as screening blood for HIV, blood and blood products are now as safe as they can be in the United Kingdom. However, it is important to remember that countries that are less wealthy may not have as good a set of screening procedures for HIV.

Someone who has a blood transfusion in a Third World country, for whatever reason, would be well advised to have an HIV test to make sure they have not been given contaminated blood. In some of these countries people are offered payment for blood donation and this, unfortunately, encourages people who are more at risk for HIV who are in need of money (to pay for drugs in many cases) to donate blood. This is why in the UK a system of voluntary donation is preferred.

There is much research into 're-using' someone's blood during operations and procedures. In this process, known as 'autologous transfusion', a person's blood is stored prior to an operation, to be given back to them during or after the operation as needed. In this way, the need for donors is avoided. There is also research into genetically engineering blood product substitutes so that blood from donors does not have to be used. This would make such supplies safer.

Organ donations, such as a kidney or liver, are also screened for HIV. Prior to a transplant operation both the donor and recipient are tested for HIV as well as other blood-borne viruses. In this situation the problem with the 'window period' remains and a small number of people have been infected post-organ transplant. Similarly semen, which is donated for artificial insemination, is also a potential risk for HIV transmission. In the past a small number of women have been infected following insemination from donors.

Nosocomial infection

Nosocomial infection occurs when HIV is passed on within a work setting, either from doctor to patient or from patient to patient or from patient to doctor. Usually, nosocomial infection occurs in the UK through accidents within the hospital such as needle-stick injuries or blood spillage. In developing countries where infrastructure and resources are limited, needles, syringes and surgical equipment are often re-used, thus resulting in further new epidemics of HIV infection.

There has been much debate in the UK as to the exact risk of transmission of HIV from a health care worker to a patient; for this reason guidelines have been drawn up with specific recommendations. Health care workers who are HIV-positive are not allowed to work in surgical settings such as operating theatres where there is a risk to the patient. They are, however, allowed to practice in other medical settings where they do not pose any more risk to the patient compared with someone who is not HIV-positive. In addition, they are required to inform their occupational health department of their HIV status and this information is confidential.

Infected health care workers should be protected themselves from placing their health at risk if their immune system is damaged. Health care workers, by and large, are at much greater risk of HIV *from* their patients than they are *to* their patients.

Vertical transmission

Vertical transmission occurs when HIV is passed on from mother to baby (see Chapters 3 and 9). In terms of HIV prevention there are several ways in which the risk of infection to the baby can be reduced. Between 13–25 per cent of children born to mothers who are HIV-positive will become infected. This figure is higher in less advantaged countries, for example, it can be 39 per cent in some African countries. The reason why this figure is not even higher is not clear and seems especially strange given the very close contact of mother with baby, through the shared circulation of blood in the mother's placenta. Unfortunately, approximately one-quarter of babies who are HIV-positive die within the first year of life.

The risk of the baby contracting HIV from the mother can be reduced in several ways; the next section focuses on mother and baby care in developed countries, in other words where real choices are available.

Breast-feeding

Breast-feeding doubles the risk of passing on HIV – therefore mothers are encouraged to bottle-feed as this is the simplest and most direct way of reducing the risk of infection from mother to baby. In developing countries, however, the recommendation is still that women should breast-feed because of the risks of other infections that are very easily passed on through poor sanitation and hygiene when bottle-feeding.

Caesarian section

The mother can be offered a Caesarian section. It seems that having a routine Caesarian section may reduce the risk of passing HIV on from mother to baby. However information about this is somewhat unclear. It is thought that a significant amount of HIV transmission occurs during the passage of the baby through the birth canal.

If the mother decides to have a normal, vaginal delivery then this should be completed as swiftly as possible with limited use of monitoring and instruments such as foetal scalp electrodes. The reason is that some of these procedures, for example the foetal scalp electrode, may cause trauma to the baby, thus increasing the risk of HIV transmission.

AZT (Zidovudine)

It has recently been discovered, after a large trial was conducted (Conner et al. 1994), that using *AZT (Zidovudine)* during the mother's pregnancy and labour, followed by use afterwards in baby will also reduce the risk of the baby becoming HIV-positive. In this study, women were either given AZT or a placebo (dummy pill). It was found that women in the AZT 'arm' of the trial had only an 8 per cent risk of transmitting HIV to their baby. For the women in the placebo 'arm' the risk was 25 per cent. This trial was stopped early as the results were so clear; in other words AZT successfully reduced the risk of transmission of HIV from mother to baby. However a number of questions remain from the design of the trial. One of the most important is that it is still unclear when AZT (Zidovudine) maximally reduces the risk of vertical transmission.

As a result of these findings, many women opt to take this drug during pregnancy. AZT is usually given throughout pregnancy starting at 14 weeks. It is suggested that women take AZT at a dose of 100 mgs five times a day, which can be quite hard to remember. AZT is not recommended in the early stages of pregnancy because women often feel nauseous anyway and may not be able to tolerate the AZT. Secondly, this is the stage when most of the major organs are developing in the baby and, although there is no evidence that AZT causes harm to the baby, it is thought best to avoid unnecessary medication at this stage.

It is recommended that women continue to receive AZT intravenously during labour, thus maintaining the medication right up until the baby is born. Then the baby is given AZT in a syrup form for six weeks after delivery. In a large study it was found that the only side-effect from giving babies AZT in this regime was that they might become mildly anaemic. This is closely monitored and can be treated.

AZT is the only drug that is licensed for use during pregnancy in the United Kingdom. Clearly, it is an effective form of treatment for the baby, as it reduces the risk of the baby being infected with HIV. Unfortunately, AZT as the single drug allowed during pregnancy is not the optimum treatment for the mother's HIV infection (see Chapter 3 for further details).

Currently, studies are being carried out looking into whether other drugs may be useful to use in combination with AZT, so that both mother and baby can receive optimal treatments. It is possible that 3TC (Lamivudine) may be safe during pregnancy but it is not yet licensed for use during pregnancy. Obviously drugs need to be deemed entirely safe before they are licensed and many of the HIV drugs are extremely new to doctors and patients. The long-term effects of these drugs are not known and caution is needed before they can be used during pregnancy. This is a rapidly evolving field of HIV medicine with information changing all the time so it is helpful for doctors and patients to keep as up to date as possible (see Chapters 3 and 8 for further details).

Thus, in many ways the risk of a baby being infected can be dramatically reduced; however, there is no guarantee – even if the mother does all of the above, there is still a small chance (5 per cent) that the baby will be infected.

HIV testing during pregnancy

Most women who are HIV-positive and pregnant in the UK are not aware of their HIV status. This was discovered by taking anonymous blood samples from pregnant women in different hospitals in the UK in order to establish how common HIV was in different settings (DOH 1995). Neither the doctors nor the women were informed of the result. A wide variation in the numbers of women who were HIV-positive was found regionally and in some parts of London it was as high as 1:200. It has been recommended in the UK that where HIV is relatively common, all pregnant women are offered the opportunity to have an HIV test during their pregnancy (Miller and Madge

1997). By identifying these women, they can be offered the various interventions discussed above to reduce the chances of their baby being infected and access treatment themselves.

Pregnancy is not an ideal time for a woman to find out that she is HIV-positive. This is especially poignant since, for some women, major decisions need to be made about the pregnancy including how the pregnancy should be managed. Medical and psychological support is available in such situations.

Ideally it would be better to test all women for HIV before they decided to become pregnant but practically this is much harder to achieve (see Chapter 8 for further details). However, the idea of having a pre-conception HIV test is extremely practical and many couples choose to do this as well as having a check-up for other sexually transmitted diseases at the same time.

Common myths about HIV transmission

HIV has been apparent for nearly twenty years; the virus itself was identified over ten years ago and most people, it is thought, are all supposedly well-educated about HIV. Unfortunately, there are still some myths about how HIV is transmitted that persist and will not go away.

It is not possible to catch HIV through saliva exchange, that is, kissing, sharing cutlery, general domestic contact or even spitting. The virus is not present in sufficient quantities in the saliva to enable it to be passed on in such a way; if it was, many more people would be infected. However, there is slight confusion in that it is now possible to test for HIV antibodies in saliva – the 'HIV test' detects antibodies to the virus and not the virus itself. The test is extremely sensitive and it is able to detect even low levels of HIV antibodies. Although saliva tests can indicate that HIV antibodies are present, it does not necessarily mean that HIV virus is present in sufficient amounts (although clearly it is present) to pose a high risk of transmission.

HIV cannot usually be passed on through contact with other body fluids such as urine or faeces. However, it is sensible to use hygienic precautions when handling such body fluids and to wear gloves wherever possible.

Some people think that HIV can be passed on through contact with sweat. This is not true.

Similarly, HIV cannot be transmitted through mosquitoes or other insects – if this *were* the case, many millions more people would be infected the world over.

Sharing razors is not recommended for people who are HIV-positive. The only way that infection could possibly occur through shaving is in the following scenario: someone who is HIV-positive cuts themselves while using a razor, to be followed by someone else who immediately picks up that same razor, who also then cuts themselves. This seems so daft as to be farcical. The main point is that sharing razors is probably not a good idea for all sorts of hygiene-related reasons.

Needle-stick injuries

A needle-stick injury occurs when someone accidentally jabs themselves with a needle or another sharp instrument which has been used on someone else. These commonly occur in hospitals but with the increasing number of procedures that can be carried out at home, these are just as likely to occur either at home or in general practitioner (GP) surgeries.

The best way to avoid a needle-stick injury is to be aware that rushing around leaves the health care worker particularly vulnerable to any sharp instruments, including needles and syringes. Experience suggests that many needle-stick injuries occur in emergency situations when people are not taking as much care as they would normally. Hence, needles or other sharp instruments should be handled with the care that they deserve.

Due care and attention should be taken; ensure that good lighting is available and that the patient is relaxed and as co-operative as possible. Gloves should be worn when dealing with blood and any open cuts should be covered with a plaster.

If a health care worker is unfortunate enough to sustain a jab from a used needle the first thing to do is to encourage bleeding. This means to squeeze the stabbed area and then as quickly as possible, the area should be cleaned with water and a disinfectant if possible. The area of skin should then be covered and contact made with the senior staff or occupational health unit for further advice. There ought to be set procedures for this type of event, especially in the larger hospital units and the big cities of the country. The general protocol for this event is as follows:

If the source person of the needle-stick injury is not known to be HIV-positive, the usual procedure is a discussion with that particular patient about an infection screen. Thus, following consent, HIV testing occurs, along with other blood-borne viruses such as hepatitis B and C.

If the source person is known and confirmed to be HIV-positive then the occupational health unit should be contacted as quickly as possible. In most hospitals people who have sustained a significant needle-stick injury from someone who is HIV-positive will now be offered triple anti-viral combination therapy, commonly AZT, 3TC and Indinavir. The drugs should be taken for one month, having started them as soon as practically possible, after the needle-stick injury, preferably within a few hours. If someone is to start on a month's triple combination treatment they need to have a reasonably lengthy discussion prior to doing this in order to clarify certain issues such as how and when the medication should be taken, any side-effects and the potential drug interactions (see Chapter 8 for details of drug regimes).

Fortunately the risk of acquiring HIV infection from a single needle-stick injury seems to be relatively small (0.2 per cent) but there have been cases of health care workers in the UK sero-converting following such injuries. It is also known that the risk of acquiring HIV from a needle-stick injury is greater if a significant injury occurs with a large-bore (or wider) needle. The risk is also greater if the source patient has advanced HIV disease or a high viral load. Such information is helpful for occupational doctors so that they can make a full assessment of risk following a needle-stick injury and consider offering post-exposure prophylaxis. Overall this means that not only do HIV doctors need to be aware of this information but also occupational health and casualty units need to be geared up to this type of arrangement. Unfortunately in other countries, where HIV is more common and resources limited, more health care workers are at risk from occupational exposure.

Blood will normally be taken for storage from the person who has acquired the needle-stick injury for purposes of testing at a later stage. This is a 'baseline' HIV test. Because of the 'window period' it will not give any information about the person's HIV status other than up to three months before the accident occurred. The person will then have subsequent bloods taken (serial blood tests) over the next three months to see if they develop HIV. Other tests may be done during this period such as a P24 antigen test and an HIV viral load which may give an earlier indication regarding HIV status.

It is important that all needle-stick injuries are reported and that procedure is followed in the described way. In the extremely unlikely event that someone contracts HIV through their work, financial compensation is more likely to be given if a stated protocol is rigorously followed.

Unfortunately, HIV is not the only virus that can be transmitted through needle-stick injuries. Hepatitis B is more infectious and anyone who is at risk from a needle-stick injury should be vaccinated against hepatitis B; indeed any clinician working with patients should be vaccinated against hepatitis B. This is also true for care workers and care assistants who are in contact with all types of patient groups.

The protection from a set of hepatitis B immunisations declines with time so it is a good idea to have blood levels of the vaccination checked every few years (usually three to five years) to make sure a booster vaccination is not needed. Other viruses, for example hepatitis C which has recently come to light, can also be transmitted through needle-stick injuries.

By following good practice procedures, needle-stick injuries can be avoided but it is important that there are contingency plans which can be implemented if accidents occur.

Travelling abroad

When travelling abroad to other countries, particularly those where HIV is more common such as Africa, India and the Far East, it is important to think about HIV prevention. Travel packs, containing sterile needles and syringes, are now available. In the unlikely event that they will need admission to hospital travellers have their own supply of clean equipment.

A much more likely scenario, however, is that people will have sex abroad, especially if they are on holiday. Packing a good supply of condoms and ample quantities of lubricant is a good idea, even if a holiday romance is not planned.

Where to test for HIV

Sexually transmitted disease (STD) clinics

There are a variety of places where someone can seek testing for HIV. Historically the most common was in a sexually transmitted disease (STD) clinic (Johnson et al. 1994). This is clearly sensible if an individual is worried that they may have put themselves at risk, in other words, they may have acquired an STD, including HIV infection. In such circumstances the STD clinic will screen for various sexually transmitted infections at the same time. There is no need to be referred to an STD clinic by a doctor. Some clinics have an appointment system and others a 'walk in' service. They often go under euphemistic names such as 'Special Clinic' or they may be called the 'Genito-Urinary Clinic' or 'Sexually Transmitted Disease Clinic'.

When HIV infection was first identified there were very few treatments available. It was thought that most people would benefit from a longer discussion or *counselling* before having a test. Historically discussions about HIV testing were up to an hour long. The thinking about this has changed quite radically: people are seeking testing more frequently, the stigma attached to HIV seems to be decreasing, albeit slowly, and there are more treatments now available for HIV infection. However, it is still recommended that a brief, focused *discussion* takes place prior to having an HIV test (DOH 1996, Miller and Lipman 1994).

If someone attends a sexually transmitted disease clinic they may have a discussion about HIV testing either with a doctor or with a health adviser. In the vast majority of cases, partly for reasons of confidentiality, clinics will insist that someone attends personally for their HIV result. This enables a discussion to take place about future behaviour and risks and also about HIV prevention if the result is negative. As the result cannot be predicted, nobody should receive a positive result over the telephone (although this has happened in the recent past).

Some special clinics can perform HIV tests on the same day. Here an individual has an appointment in the morning and a discussion about the HIV test. The result is then available in the afternoon.

Alternatives to testing at STD clinics

As time has gone on it has been realised that some people may not access a sexually transmitted disease clinic. They may not wish to go there – unfortunately some stigma does remain – or they may not feel that the clinic is the appropriate place for the test. It is important therefore that other settings are able to offer HIV tests, where suitably qualified clinicians can initiate the appropriate discussions about lifestyle, risk and prevention of HIV infection in an atmosphere which is non-judgmental, private and confidential.

Many general practitioners (GPs) will carry out HIV tests, if requested by their patients, or to exclude HIV infection as a cause for symptoms. Some people prefer to discuss HIV testing with their GP if they have a good relationship with them. They may have discussed previous risks with them at prior consultations.

Much has been made in the past about future life insurance concerns even if someone's test is HIV-negative. This is becoming less and less of a problem nowadays. The British Association of Insurers has recommendations that specify information about negative HIV tests need *not* be disclosed and they are only seeking information regarding those who have tested HIV-positive (Association of British Insurers 1994). Therefore people should not be dissuaded from having a test with their general practitioner or elsewhere in other hospital settings. The British Medical Association (BMA) recommends that no specific questions about lifestyle or sexual orientation are answered by GPs on insurance forms. In fact many GPs are using a previously agreed statement which states that 'in accordance with BMA guidelines such lifestyle questions are not speculated upon' (see Chapter 6 for further details). Hence in the future it is likely that an increased variety of settings will be offering HIV tests. This is especially critical as HIV can be very non-specific in its presentation. People with early HIV infection may present to different hospital settings with symptoms relating to HIV.

They may therefore be asked to consider HIV testing to exclude this as a differential diagnosis.

Hospital services may also offer HIV tests when they are considering HIV as part of a differential diagnosis. Other settings are increasingly offering HIV testing as part of a screening procedure, especially in areas of the UK where HIV is common, for example, pregnant women are routinely being offered HIV testing in London to enable them to be offered methods of reducing vertical transmission (see Chapter 9).

Finally, there are also private clinics that will offer rapid HIV test results. The quality of discussion, prior to and after testing, in these clinics may vary, and a fee is charged.

Consent to HIV testing

No one should be coerced into having an HIV test. HIV testing should always be carried out with the consent of the individual. There are some settings where people are routinely tested for HIV, such as when donating blood or prior to organ donation.

Unfortunately, in the past some people have had HIV tests performed without their consent. When this occurs, especially if the result comes back HIV-positive, it is obviously extremely shocking and distressing for the individual concerned. This is extremely bad practice and most probably 'illegal'. Quite simply this should *never* happen nowadays.

Testing without consent is also bad practice because full evaluation of risks, (for example the window period) cannot be made. No discussion about future risks and HIV prevention can occur and thus is a fairly pointless exercise and a lost opportunity to discuss HIV prevention.

In a few settings HIV testing is mandatory, for example, when applying for visas or citizenship in certain countries. Only those who are tested HIV-negative are allowed to enter these countries. The embassies of these countries provide HIV testing facilities. However, communication from those who have been tested in this way suggests the service provided can be very variable. Some people choose to seek testing at an alternative site if a full discussion about risks and future prevention is preferred.

The authors feel that it is important that a doctor is present when someone is given an HIV-positive result. Historically, in some settings, this has not always been the case, and counsellors have taken on this role. Probably the best working arrangement, where resources are sufficient, is that both counsellor and doctor are present. Many patients may have questions of a medical nature pertaining to HIV infection and it is beneficial to have a doctor present to answer these. Also some people have a test when they are unwell and a full medical assessment may be necessary to exclude any serious life-threatening infection at that time. For most people, receiving an HIV-positive result is extremely stressful. A small number of people may express suicidal ideas. In this case it is prudent to have a doctor at hand in order to clinically assess the physical and emotional state of the individual before accessing further help if necessary.

HIV prevention – what strategies work?

As yet, the best way to encourage people to use safer sex remains unclear. In other words, what strategies are most effective in promoting safer sex are unknown, though there are many research projects which have tried to tackle this problem. National campaigns can raise general awareness and education in schools for children at a young age is also vitally important. However, personal experience of HIV is likely to be the most effective strategy in terms of HIV prevention. Some health professionals think that until people come into direct contact with HIV through friends, family or partners they may not question their own behaviour.

Many people in the UK are at extremely low risk of HIV and it is very unlikely that in their lifetime they will have any contact of any sort with someone who is HIV-positive. Other people are much more at risk. One individual's personal strategy for HIV prevention may be quite different to another person's. Whatever approach is adopted, advice and information should be accessible to help people make decisions.

References

Association of British Insurers (1994) *ABI Statement of Practice – Underwriting Life Insurance for HIV/AIDS*, Association of British Insurers, 51 Gresham Street, London EC2 7HQ.

Connor, E.M., Sperling, R.S., Gelber, R. et al. (1994) 'Reduction in maternal infant transmission of human immunodeficiency virus type I with Zidovudine treatment', *New England Journal of Medicine*, 331: 1173–80.

DOH (1992) *Guidelines for offering voluntary HIV antibody testing to women receiving ante-natal care*, London: Department of Health.

DOH, Unlinked Anonymous HIV Surveys Steering Group (1996) 'Unlinked anonymous HIV prevalence monitoring programme: England and Wales, Data to the end of 1995', London: Department of Health, Public Health Laboratory Services, Institute of Child Health.

DOH (1996) *Guidelines for pre-test discussion on HIV testing*, London: Department of Health (DOH).

Gill, O.N., Noone, A. and Heptonstall, J. (1995) 'Imprisonment, injecting drug use and blood borne viruses', *British Medical Journal*, 310: 275–6.

Gore, S.M., Bird, G., Burns, S.M. et al. (1995) 'Drug injection and HIV prevalence in inmates of Glenochil prison', *British Medical Journal*, 310: 293–6.

Grosskurth, H., Mosha, F., Mwijarubi, E. et al. (1995) 'Impact of improved treatment of sexually transmitted diseases on HIV infection in rural Tanzania: A randomised controlled trial', *Lancet*, 340: 530–6.

Johnson, A.M., Wadsworth, J., Wellings, K. et al. (1994) *Sexual attitudes and lifestyle*, Oxford: Blackwell Scientific Publications.

Miller R. and Lipman, M. (1996) 'HIV pre-test discussion', *British Medical Journal*, 313: 130.

Miller R. and Madge, S. (1997) 'Routine HIV testing in antenatal care, time to move on', *The Diplomate*, 4: 26–31.

3 The Natural History of HIV Infection

The clinical manifestations of human immuno-deficiency (HIV) infection have been divided into different stages and we aim to describe these in this section. There are, however, important points that need to be mentioned first.

When exactly an individual decides to be tested for HIV infection is extremely variable and influenced by many different factors. This means that someone may be diagnosed early on in the course of the disease, or later on if and when symptoms develop, or when they develop AIDS. It is therefore clear that there is often little correlation between how long a person has been aware of their diagnosis and the development of symptoms. Some people may know when they were likely to have been infected from their risk behaviour.

Second, the course of HIV disease in different people varies tremendously and to some extent is unpredictable. Factors thought to have a role include:

- The specific individual immune response evoked by the infection
- The age of the person infected (older people tend to do worse)
- The strain of HIV itself (discussed in this chapter)
- If the person who was the source of the infection was on anti-viral medication, as resistance to medication may be important
- Other genetic factors.

In addition, people cope with HIV infection in many different ways. Factors which influence how people cope include family or social support, a person's psychological state as well as the individual's beliefs and spiritual standing.

Finally, HIV infection can affect every part of the body, from the skin to various internal organs such as the lungs, the gastro-intestinal tract and the neurological system. Sometimes HIV infection can result in a wide variety of seemingly unrelated symptoms. However, it is also important to remember that any individual who is HIV-positive can suffer other illnesses and ailments that are not related to their HIV infection. In other words, it is tempting to blame HIV infection for all the problems the person is experiencing.

Some basic guidelines for healthy living

Before describing the various stages of HIV infection, it is prudent to note some basic 'healthy living' guidelines that may be beneficial to those individuals at risk of or with HIV infection and are good guides to a healthy lifestyle generally.

Eating a healthy, balanced diet

There has been considerable work on different types of diet in people with HIV infection. However, there is little evidence that any particular stringent diet confers benefit over another diet with regards to HIV infection. Some people choose a strict exclusion diet, however some of these may not provide adequate number of calories or even an adequate nutrient content. Some people may end up spending unnecessary amounts of time and money on special unproved diets. A dietician is always a good source of advice and guidance on this subject is generally a good idea, especially if someone is starting medication, as there are often requirements around food and HIV medication (see Chapters 4 and 8).

Exercise and physical activity

There is good evidence to show that exercise is important for a number of reasons. Exercise can reduce stress and often helps people to feel better. In addition, physical activity improves muscle bulk and may help to reduce weight loss in those who are suffering intercurrent illness. Even in the latter stages of HIV infection, simple exercises are possible that can help a person's quality of life. Physiotherapists are often keen to discuss exercise programmes with patients and some gyms have special provision for those with HIV infection (see Chapter 6).

Smoking

Many people decide when they have been diagnosed HIV-positive that they will try to give up smoking and this is to be encouraged. There is some evidence that smoking is harmful to the immune system and it can increase the chance of chest infections, which are invariably more common in those with HIV infection. As people live longer with HIV a 'long-term' view of their health should be adopted and stopping smoking is important in reducing heart disease, chest problems and cancers. It seems that lung cancer is becoming more common in people with HIV, though the reason for this is unclear.

Alcohol

Alcohol in moderation is fine (and recommended). However, in excess, alcohol is harmful and this is particularly the case in those with previous liver infections such as hepatitis B or C. Advice and guidance can be obtained from health education leaflets, clinicians and nursing staff. The guidance given by most doctors is that 21 units a week in men and 14 units a week in women are the maximum safe amounts. A unit is half a pint of beer or lager or a normal-sized glass of wine or one measure of spirits.

Recreational drugs

Many people choose to use recreational drugs either regularly or intermittently. Many of these may be harmful to the immune system as well as to health in general. Specialist advice is available from drug projects, clinicians or special drug workers.

Safer sex

If a person has been diagnosed HIV-positive it is important to practice safer sex, not only to reduce the risk of transmission to others, but also to prevent acquiring other sexually transmitted diseases. Any sexually transmitted disease in a person with HIV infection can be more persistent and thus more difficult to treat.

In addition, there is evidence that Kaposi's sarcoma, a well-recognised AIDS-related tumour, may be sexually transmitted (see later this chapter). As HIV is viewed as a more treatable condition there is increasing concern that more people will be prepared to take increased risks by having unsafe sex. There is some evidence that this is happening in the UK especially in young gay men. One possible consequence of this is that as more people are on HIV treatments and the virus is able to become resistant to these drugs, people who are newly infected with HIV will 'inherit' resistant virus. Drug treatments in these people may therefore be less effective.

Seroconversion (primary HIV infection)

When a person is infected with the HIV virus they may have what is called a 'seroconversion illness'. The majority of people with HIV infection will at least experience some symptoms during the time that they are becoming HIV-positive, but the range of symptoms and the degree to which a particular person is affected is very broad. Typically these symptoms occur a few weeks after the person has been exposed to HIV. Many people will present to their general practitioner (GP) and a small number, who may be aware of their risk for HIV, may attend specialist services for diagnosis and possible treatment. Unfortunately, the symptoms of the seroconversion illness are fairly non-specific as are most flu-like illnesses. Therefore, if people present with such symptoms to their GP, HIV as a potential diagnosis, is often not considered. The following symptoms may occur during the seroconversion period:

- Tiredness
- Sweats and fever
- Muscle aches
- Joint pains
- Mouth ulcers and genital ulcers
- Headache (particularly behind the eyes)
- A fine red rash over the trunk of the body
- Nausea, vomiting and diarrhoea
- Swollen lymph glands.

Symptoms of a seroconversion illness classically appear between two and six weeks after exposure to the HIV risk. These symptoms may last from a few days to many weeks, but some people will not experience any symptoms at all. A small number of people may have a more marked seroconversion illness and be more severely unwell and may have neurological features. This is, however, rare.

When someone is having a seroconversion illness the HIV antibody test may be positive, negative or in-between. This is because, during this phase, the body is producing HIV antibodies and at the time they have the test there may or may not be sufficient antibodies to register a positive result. Therefore any one who has had a risk for HIV within three months of seeking an HIV test is advised to have a repeat test if the initial test is negative as they are in this 'window period' of potential antibody production.

For people who may be aware that they have recently put themselves at risk from HIV there are more special tests that can be done to establish the diagnosis of acute HIV infection at an early stage. These may include tests such as HIV viral load and p24 antigen. However, these can only be done in special hospital settings and would not be generally available through general practice.

Among doctors, there is a lot of interest in seroconversion illness. In studies carried out in the United States and Europe, a small number of people who were diagnosed during their seroconversion illness have been given three anti-HIV drugs. They are being very closely followed up to see whether HIV may be eradicated from their bodies or, if their outcome could be improved by having such early treatment. In the UK, if someone is definitely diagnosed as having been very recently infected with HIV, doctors may well suggest that they think about starting on anti-viral drugs. However, there is a lot of uncertainty in starting such treatment. There is no guarantee that it will improve their outcome, they may well have side-effects and it is unclear when doctors should stop such treatment in these circumstances. However, it is thought that such studies are important if further lessons are to be learnt about the natural history of HIV infection and thus to find potential ways of treating or curing it.

Asymptomatic HIV disease

Following seroconversion with HIV, an individual may then be very well with no major symptoms at all for many years. The only way to diagnose HIV infection in such people is for them to have an HIV antibody test. There are no other tests that would tell whether someone had HIV infection and there would be no specific signs or symptoms to look out for.

Symptomatic HIV disease

As the HIV virus manages to compromise the immune system people may develop minor symptoms that are related to HIV. Because these are often minor, non-specific and may be self-limiting, they are often missed by clinicians, including doctors in the community and the hospital. Most of these symptoms are easy to treat. HIV primarily affects lymphocytes, cells which make up the white blood cell population and which especially fight and protect against viral and fungal infections. Therefore, it is not surprising that many of the symptoms someone with HIV has are due to viral and fungal infections. These symptoms increase in frequency generally as the number of T cells and lymphocytes decrease with HIV advancing disease. Some of the more common symptoms are discussed below (Adler 1993,

Mindel and Miller 1996, Lipman et al. 1993).

Skin problems

A number of skin-related conditions are more common in people who are HIV positive. These include:

- Shingles (herpes zoster) is often more serious in people who are HIV-positive and is caused by the herpes virus that causes chicken pox. Someone can only get shingles if they have already had chicken pox, though it is possible to 'catch' chicken pox from someone who has shingles. A rash appears in a certain distribution on one part of the body and may be itchy, with blisters and can be quite painful. Shingles can affect any part of the body.
  It is especially common and dangerous on the face, because of the potential to cause scarring to the surface of the eye. People who have shingles that affects the eye need to be seen by an eye specialist for review and follow-up. However, shingles is easily treated by a course of treatment with aciclovir or Famvir. A small number of people may get nasty pain from damage to the nerve endings following shingles that can be problematic to treat. Drugs such as carbamazepine or amytriptyline can be used.
- Warts are more common in people with HIV disease and can be treated in the usual way often with freezing therapy (cryotherapy).
- Dry skin is more common with HIV disease and is treated with bath emollients and aqueous cream. These need to be used regularly. Dry skin can often be quite itchy. Some people find that biological washing powders can worsen dry skin, so non-biological ones are preferred.
- Psoriasis can be quite severe in people with HIV disease and is treated in the usual way.
- Eczema is also common.
- Folliculitis is inflammation of the hair follicles, causing small red spots on the body; this can be treated by cleaning the body with surgical scrub and occasionally may need courses of antibiotics.
- Scabies can be more common and difficult to treat in people with HIV disease. It is caused by a mite which burrows under the skin and is very infectious to anyone who may come in contact with someone who is infected. Multiple treatments with malathion lotion may be necessary.
- Molluscum contagiosum is caused by a pox virus and causes raised pearly lesions often on the face and upper body. They can be spread by shaving and are best treated with cryotherapy in the same way as warts.

● Seborrheic dermatitis is a fungal infection that typically appears along the centre of the face. It can be treated with anti-fungal cream like Canestan. It can also affect the scalp and special shampoos can help.
● Fungal nail infections are also common and may need treatment with a drug called terbinafine, sometimes for up to six months. Other fungal infections are also more common, such as athlete's foot.

Genital infections

Genital infections are more common in people with HIV:

● Thrush (candida) is especially common in women and may be an early sign of damage to the immune system. It can be treated with Canestan pessaries or fluconazole tablets which can now be bought from pharmacists without a prescription.
● Recurrent herpes infections can be problematic in men and women with HIV disease and may need long-term preventative treatment with aciclovir.
● Genital warts need treating either with topical paints that are applied locally or freezing (cryotherapy). A consequence of genital warts in women is that they are more likely to have abnormal smears. Women with HIV are advised to have more frequent cervical (PAP) smears than women who are not known to be HIV-positive.

Other sexually transmitted diseases such as chlamydia or gonorrhoea are only likely to occur if someone is not using condoms. Most HIV treatment centres offer regular screening for sexually transmitted diseases for people who are HIV-positive. This is important because many sexually transmitted diseases are asymptomatic and it is also known that other STDs increase the risk of HIV being transmitted.

Oral infections

The mouth is a common site for HIV-related problems and dentists may often identify such problems and suggest that people have an HIV test. Common HIV-related oral problems include:

● Thrush is a common infection in the mouth. It can cause a sore throat or painful areas at the corners of the mouth. Thrush typically causes white rounded areas in the mouth, especially at the back of the throat. It can be treated by various drugs such as itraconazole, fluconazole or Nystatin pastilles. Thrush may cause more painful symptoms if it is present further down the mouth in the oesophagus (food pipe or gullet), where it might cause discomfort on swallowing. Oral thrush can be precipitated in anyone irrespective of their HIV status, for example, following a recent course of antibiotics or if someone is using a steroid inhaler for asthma.

- Oral hairy leukoplakia is a sign of the immune system being damaged. It presents with small white plaques on the side of the tongue. These may look like fine hairs, hence the name, and may come and go. The condition does not usually need any specific treatment itself. Classically it is supposed to be asymptomatic; however, anecdotally a minority of people complain of tenderness and pain on the sides of the tongue.
- Cold sores are caused by the herpes virus and can be treated with aciclovir cream or tablets.
- Aphthous ulcers are more common in people with HIV and can be quite problematic to treat. Adcortyl in orabase paste may be used or Corlan pellets.
- Gingivitis, inflammation of the gums, may need treatment with mouthwash or courses of antibiotics such as metronidazole.

Many of these conditions can be to some degree prevented, hence people with HIV are advised to see dentists for regular check-ups and advice (see Chapter 6).

Additional signs and symptoms of HIV

Other non-specific symptoms and signs of HIV disease include:

- Lymphadenopathy are areas of swollen, sometimes painful, lymph glands commonly in the neck, under the arms and in the groin. The lymph nodes are the clearing sites for the body to deal with infection. The swellings may come and go over a period of months and are especially common in people with HIV disease.
- Diarrhoea may be intermittent and may respond well to simple treatment such as loperamide or codeine phosphate. If diarrhoea is persistent, it needs investigating to exclude any infectious cause.
- Night sweats and lethargy are common symptoms of HIV disease and can be very difficult to treat. Sometimes when a person starts on anti-viral treatments these symptoms often improve. Night sweats can be very debilitating. Sweats in general can also occur also during the day, but more frequently at night necessitating change of night clothes and sheets. Paracetamol and aspirin may help, as well as some of the other

non-steroidal drugs such as Naproxen. Sweats are very common in people with HIV infection but may also be a sign of other illnesses that are more common in people with HIV, such as tuberculosis (TB) and lymphomas.

- Tiredness is probably the most common symptom of which people with HIV infection complain. It is not surprising given than anyone with a chronic viral infection may well complain of this symptom. As many GPs know, feeling 'tired all the time' is a frequent complaint of the general population. However, it should not be dismissed or underestimated and other causes should be investigated. Sometimes when someone is depressed they may feel tired. It may also be a function of not sleeping, for whatever reason. Anaemia may also present with tiredness as may other unrelated conditions such as diabetes or reduced thyroid function. In a person with HIV infection, tiredness and lethargy can often be reversed dramatically on starting anti-viral treatments.

- Sinusitis and ear infections are more common in people with HIV disease and often need treatment with antibiotics. Other treatments that may be helpful in sinusitis include steroid nasal sprays which can reduce the recurrence rate of sinusitis if used regularly. Simple inhalation with steam two or three times a day can provide temporary, but often dramatic, symptomatic relief.

- People with HIV are often more sensitive to drug treatments such as antibiotics and may be more likely to have drug reactions and allergies.

This is not intended to be an exhaustive list of every symptom that someone with HIV may experience. Some people may be fortunate and only have these symptoms to a minor degree. Others are less lucky. Many of these common symptoms can be managed in general practice but it is important that hospital doctors know the sort of symptoms someone has been experiencing as they are often markers of the immune system becoming more damaged.

AIDS

AIDS is the acronym for Acquired Immune Deficiency Syndrome. It is composed of a group of illnesses that may occur in the presence of HIV and are described as 'AIDS-defining'. AIDS-related problems consist of *opportunistic infections*, that is, many HIV/AIDS-related infections are fairly common, but in people with normal immune systems they tend not to cause so many problems. However, if someone has a very damaged immune system, for example in HIV or advanced AIDS, then these same infections often cause different and severe symptoms (Adler 1993, Mindel and Miller 1996, Lipman et al. 1993). AIDS illnesses are often viral or fungal infections in keeping with having a depleted lymphocyte count. In the UK CD4 count does not determine whether or not you have AIDS unlike in the US, where a CD4 count of below 200 is the indicator for AIDS.

Most acute AIDS-related problems need to be treated in hospital. Often they can be treated very successfully and it is not uncommon for someone to experience several of the major AIDS-related diseases. Unfortunately there is no way of predicting which people are likely to get which AIDS-related problems.

As the result of extensive research over the past 15 years in HIV and AIDS, several major AIDS-related infections can be prevented with simple treatments. In fact this has been so successful that some infections and conditions are becoming less common. Moreover, with the use of the newer combination anti-viral treatments, there does seem to be a change in the diseases that are most common. For example, cytomegalovirus (CMV) disease is becoming much less common than in the past (see later this chapter).

The list of AIDS-related diseases below is not intended to be exhaustive but refers to the most common diseases that occur.

TB (tuberculosis)

TB usually affects the lungs, but can affect the lymph nodes, gastro-intestinal tract, brain and other parts of the body. It is more common in people with HIV disease. It often presents when people have reasonably good immune systems compared to the other AIDS-related illnesses, that is, when their CD4 counts are around 200 or 300. TB is more common in people who come from developing countries, those who have injected drugs and the homeless. Treatment is generally the same regardless of HIV status. The treatment involves several antibiotics for many months and often people will stay on at least two antibiotics to prevent the TB from coming back in the future. People who are particularly at risk from TB may be offered what is called prophylactic treatment, frequently a drug called isoniazid to reduce the chances of them getting the disease in the first place.

Common symptoms of 'active' TB include a cough with bloody sputum (haemoptysis), shortness of breath, weight loss and sweats. Most people respond well to TB treatment and often do not need to be admitted to hospital. TB is infectious and if the TB organism is found in the phlegm it may then be easily passed on to others. People who are found to have TB are 'contact traced': anyone who has been in close contact with the person with TB will be advised by a special nurse, given a check-up and may be offered preventative treatments.

Because TB is infectious to other people it presents a public health hazard and it is for this reason that specific trained nurses will become involved in contact tracing. Most people with TB are compliant with taking the antibiotics needed to clear the infection. However, in a small number of cases for a variety of reasons, some people may be less compliant. In these instances specially trained professionals such as nurses or pharmacists may be asked to participate in 'directly observed therapy' (DOT): the patient takes their medication in the presence of the nurse/pharmacist to ensure that compliance occurs.

Unfortunately, in recent years a form of TB has developed which is resistant to the usual antibiotics. This is extremely serious, but fortunately quite rare in the UK, though well-known outbreaks have occurred in some of the larger cities like London. This form of the infection is called 'multi-resistant TB'. There have been sporadic cases in the UK, but it is more common in the US.

PCP (pneumocystis carinii pneumonia)

PCP, pneumocystis carinii pneumonia, is caused by a fungal organism and was very common in people with HIV. Nowadays, it is easily prevented so it is less common. PCP is most often seen in people who are unaware of their HIV status and therefore such patients present to clinics or doctors with the acute pneumonia which is then identified as PCP. People who have damaged immune systems for other reasons, for example, those who have had organ transplants, are also at high risk of PCP. Here the immune system has been deliberately weakened by drugs to make the body less likely to reject the transplanted organ.

PCP is important because it is easily prevented. If someone has an immune system that is damaged and a CD4 count of around 200 they will generally be offered prophylactic (preventative) treatment against PCP which is highly effective.

Septrin (Co-trimoxazole) is the antibiotic that is given to most people. It is made up of two different antibiotic constituents, trimethoprim and sulphamethaxazole. One tablet a day or one tablet on alternate days will very effectively prevent PCP and also protects people from toxoplasmosis and other bacterial infections. If someone is allergic to Septrin then they may be offered alternative treatment such as pentamidine. This is given in a nebuliser form and inhaled through a mask on a monthly basis and can be done at home. Some people who are only mildly allergic to Septrin can have a Septrin desensitisation course, but this is usually under fairly close medical supervision. The desensitisation course starts with Septrin at a very low dose, which is built up over a week to the full dose of Septrin. In this way some people who are allergic to Septrin can tolerate the antibiotic.

If someone is unaware of their HIV status or has chosen not to take prophylactic treatment for PCP they may develop this disease. Common symptoms include shortness of breath, a dry cough, difficulty in taking a deep breath, fever and tiredness. Often symptoms go on for several weeks or months before someone seeks help or the seriousness of the situation is appreciated. Further tests such as a chest x-ray may also help in making the diagnosis of PCP pneumonia, though the chest x-ray can be normal if the infection is in its early stages. Another simple test for PCP is to measure the oxygen saturation of the blood before and after exercise. This is easily and painlessly done by using a special clip and probe which is attached to a finger. Sometimes to investigate symptoms further and to confirm the diagnosis of PCP a *bronchoscopy* is performed: a fine tube is passed through the nose and into the lungs and samples of fluid are taken to look for PCP. It is relatively painless and can be performed as a day case in most hospitals. A light sedative is often given to make this procedure more tolerable.

If someone is thought to have PCP pneumonia they are usually admitted to hospital and treated with intravenous Septrin via a drip. There are alternative treatments available if someone is allergic to Septrin. If they have more severe PCP they may also be given steroid treatment and oxygen via a mask. Most people with PCP are in hospital for two to three weeks. In extreme cases where PCP is very severe, a person may be very unwell and may need help with their breathing with artificial ventilation. However, this is unusual, especially if the pneumonia is identified early and treated quickly.

Toxoplasmosis

Toxoplasmosis is a protozoan infection that is less common now in people with AIDS, due to the use of Septrin which protects against toxoplasmosis as well as PCP. The infection is caused by reactivation of the toxoplasmosis organism. Many people have probably encountered toxoplasma before, usually in childhood. However because it lies dormant in the body, any reduction in functioning of the immune system may result in reactivation of this particular infection. A common source of the initial infection is via cat litter or by eating partially cooked meats. For the latter reason the disease is more common in France.

In people with HIV, toxoplasmosis can cause brain abscesses and people with toxoplasmosis may present to doctors in a variety of different ways. These include epileptic fits, confusion, erratic changes in behaviour, or even weakness down one side of their body – similar to that suffered in a stroke. Although toxoplasmosis commonly affects the brain it may also cause abscesses in different areas of the body such as the lungs. Effective treatment for toxoplasmosis is usually in the form of a drip. Drugs used include sulphadiazine, pyrimethamine, clindamycin and folinic acid (see Chapter 8). Some people are allergic to these drugs and alternatives are available such as atovoquone. Once someone has had toxoplasmosis they need to carry on with preventative treatment because there is a risk of reactivation. However, in most cases it can be successfully treated.

CMV (cytomegalovirus)

Cytomegalovirus is a common cause of AIDS-related problems. It arises from the group of herpes viruses. Again, like toxoplasmosis, CMV is a common, usually minor, illness; it is especially common in sexually active people as it is spread through saliva. It becomes a major problem when the immune system is compromised and the virus is 'reactivated'. For example, people who have had organ transplants suffer greatly with CMV-related disease as well as those who are HIV-positive. CMV may affect other organs of the body such as the stomach, colon, the brain and adrenal glands. Treatment in these cases usually involves a course of intravenous ganciclovir or foscarnet.

In people with HIV, the most worrying manifestations is CMV in the eye, something called 'CMV retinitis'. A small number of people may go blind as a result of CMV retinitis, although this usually happens if it is diagnosed late. However, it is much more common that vision may be impaired permanently. CMV disease is especially common in people with very damaged immune systems – usually their CD4 counts are below 100. It may present with only minor symptoms such as blurred vision, 'floaters' (dark specks in front of the eyes which appear to float about the visual field) or loss of part of one visual field. Therefore doctors usually look at the back of the eyes of those at risk of CMV disease in an attempt at early identification. Often too, the HIV doctors may ask the eye specialists to have a more detailed look at the retina at the back of the eye. In these circumstances special drops are put into the eye to temporarily dilate the pupil so a closer and better view is obtained.

Treatment for CMV disease is changing. In the past people needed to have continual drip treatment every day with a drug such as ganciclovir or foscarnet. This meant that they had to have a permanent intravenous access site which often led to complications such as infections and was a very intrusive and labour-intensive way of treating CMV disease. Effective oral forms of ganciclovir are now available. Other intravenous treatments (such as Cidovofir) only need to be given once every two weeks. Implants of drugs such as ganciclovir can be placed in the eye by a small operation and these may be very effective treatments. Many research projects are trying to identify people who are at greatest risk from CMV disease, in order that they may be offered treatment before actually developing the disease, thus reducing their risk of visual and other problems.

Kaposi's sarcoma (KS)

Kaposi's sarcoma is a skin tumour that arises from the lining of the blood vessels. It causes raised purple areas on the skin that can be very disfiguring. Kaposi's sarcoma, first described over 100 years ago by a dermatologist named Kaposi, can affect individuals that are HIV-negative. In its original form it had a distinct geographical distribution and is especially common in people from eastern Europe and the Mediterranean areas. In people who are HIV-negative it tends to be a more indolent disease. When HIV was discovered in the early 1980s many people presented with a different type of Kaposi's sarcoma which became associated with HIV infection.

Kaposi's sarcoma is usually diagnosed by its appearance or, occasionally, a skin biopsy. Treatment involves local radiotherapy or local chemotherapy or simply camouflaging the spots and is often very effective. Kaposi's sarcoma lesions may also disappear when people are on effective anti-viral treatment for HIV. More seriously, KS can affect the internal organs and it is especially common in the lungs and the gut. In such cases or when skin areas are very badly affected, people may need to have intravenous chemotherapy every two to three weeks.

It is thought that Kaposi's sarcoma in people with HIV is sexually transmitted; KS is very uncommon in people who are HIV-positive through drug use or blood products. The appearance of Kaposi's sarcoma may be related to one of the herpes group of viruses because epidemiological studies have shown it to have an 'infective component'. In other words a virus probably acts to 'trigger' the development of Kaposi's sarcoma in susceptible people with HIV infection. As people now have adopted safer sex practices than those of 10–20 years ago, Kaposi's sarcoma is less common than when HIV was initially discovered.

Lymphomas

Lymphomas are tumours of the lymphatic system and are unfortunately more common in people with HIV disease. Presenting as large swollen lymph nodes in the neck, under the arm or in the groin, lymphomas may also present as tumours in the brain. The ear, nose and throat area, the lungs and the gut may also be affected. Sometimes people will have non-specific symptoms such as fevers, weight loss and tiredness.

A small operation is usually performed in order to obtain body tissues for microscopic examination. This is necessary for diagnosis of a lymphoma as the symptoms are similar to TB and HIV itself. Treatment involves rigorous chemotherapy and also sometimes radiotherapy. In people who are weakened with other AIDS-related problems, this can be precarious. However, some people with lymphomas successfully tolerate the full course of treatment and thus may be cured.

AIDS-related diarrhoea

AIDS-related diarrhoea can be caused by a variety of organisms, such as microsporidium and cryptosporidium. Diarrhoea is also a common symptom in HIV itself. Other minor infections causing diarrhoea, such as giardia, are also more common in HIV; these need to be identified as treatment is different. The simplest investigation is laboratory examination of a stool sample. Often many samples need to be sent to the laboratory before the organism is found. Occasionally biopsies from the gut are taken to help make a diagnosis – this is relatively simple and can be done as an outpatient procedure.

In AIDS-related diarrhoea symptomatic treatment with drugs such as loperamide or codeine can be very effective if symptoms are only minor. If symptoms are more significant then stronger drugs such as morphine may be used. There are some antibiotics that are particularly effective against microsporidium and a short course of these may help the diarrhoea to settle.

Cryptococcal meningitis

Cryptococcal meningitis is caused by a fungal infection and often presents with a slow onset of headache, temperatures, tiredness, photophobia (painful light sensitivity) and weight loss. It is diagnosed by lumbar puncture, where the cryptococcal organism can be identified. A lumbar puncture, where a sample of fluid is taken from the spine, is a relatively simple procedure but can result in a nasty headache for a day or so after. Because of the risk of headache after the lumbar puncture, doctors advise that the patient should remain flat for several hours after.

Treatment of cryptococcal meningitis usually involves intravenous treatment with amphotericin or flucytosine for many weeks. To prevent the cryptococcal organism returning people need to take other anti-fungal treatments such as fluconazole or itraconazole tablets for the rest of their lives. Treatment can be very effective if a diagnosis of cryptococcal meningitis is made early.

Progressive multifocal leuko-encephalopathy (PML)

PML is a progressive neurological disease that can present in many different ways. Unfortunately there is no established treatment although new treatments are on trial. PML is caused by a virus known as the 'JC' virus, which may cause the patient to become progressively weaker and immobile. PML is diagnosed by its clinical course, brain scans and looking for the JC virus in a fluid sample from a lumbar puncture. The focus in many cases is on palliative care and the prognosis is very poor. Fortunately it is relatively rare.

Mycobacterium avium intracellulare (MAI)

MAI is an atypical TB-like organism. It is not infectious to other people but it is relatively common in those people with HIV with very low CD4 counts. It can present very non-specifically with weight loss, fevers, sweats and is diagnosed by taking special blood cultures. Treatment involves a complicated course of antibiotics which may often be very effective.

As more and more effective anti-viral treatments are being used, many of the 'minor' symptoms of HIV infection are becoming less common. Some of the AIDS-related illnesses too are less frequent such as PCP and CMV disease. Indeed the natural history of HIV infection seems to be changing in the presence of more effective anti-viral HIV treatment.

Women and HIV infection

The management of women with HIV is no different from men. However, a few important points should be considered (Johnson and Johnstone 1993). The prognosis for women with HIV infection is no different from that of men. World-wide, the proportion of women with HIV is increasing and is approaching that of men. However, in the UK, women make up a smaller proportion (15%) of those infected. Specific points worth stating include the fact that cervical smears are more likely to be abnormal in women with HIV infection, who are therefore recommended to have cervical smears taken every six months. Women are also more likely to develop other serious genital infections. Therefore, it is important that women who are diagnosed with HIV have close follow-up with gynaecology services.

Contraception is an important issue for many women. Condoms are preferred to reduce HIV transmission and to give protection from other sexually transmitted diseases. However, as previously stated, condoms can split or burst. Therefore, many women choose to have a double form of protection and may either take the combined contraceptive pill or have a Depo injection to provide added protection. The latter is an injection given every three months and is an effective hormonal contraceptive. It does sometimes have side-effects, such as heavy periods or, in other cases, a complete cessation of menstruating. However, if it suits a woman, it is an easy method of contraception as it does not entail remembering to take pills every day. It is probably not a good idea for women with HIV infection to have the intra-uterine coil (IUCD) as their form of contraception because of the increased risk of pelvic infections.

Discussions around future pregnancies are important and a non-judgmental, flexible attitude is essential in those caring for women with HIV infection. Many women choose to seek pregnancy and need support during this time. If a women is HIV-positive and her partner is also HIV-positive then unprotected sex at the time when one is most likely to conceive may be the best method of conception. It is somewhat more problematic when the partner is HIV-negative. In this case there are alternatives. The artificial insemination procedure, using the partners' sperm, can be relatively easily taught to women and in this circumstance the male partner is not put at risk from HIV infection. Providing the women is ovulating, this is a successful technique. Some women do choose, however, to have unprotected sex. If they are going to do this it is best to advise on the time of maximal conception so the male partner is put at as little risk as possible.

If the male partner is HIV-positive and the female partner is HIV-negative then it is a little bit more complicated. Again, unprotected sex at the time of maximal conception may be an alternative although this does put the woman at risk of contracting HIV. In Italy there has been some success with a technique called 'sperm washing', though this technique has not been validated in the UK. It does appear to have had some success and would seem to be less risky than having unprotected sex.

The situation becomes more problematic when conception is desired but does not seem to be possible. There are no specific recommendations as to how far to investigate women who are HIV-positive but appear to be sub-fertile. Most hospitals will offer investigations in the normal way to try and pinpoint exactly what the problem is and if it can be overcome. In a small number of cases, assisted conception, usually *in vitro* fertilisation (IVF), would appear to be the only way that conception may occur. HIV-positive women have been referred for IVF but the readiness and accessibility of such services is not widespread. Hopefully, in the future, guidelines and recommendations in the UK will be clearer, especially in the light of the improved prognosis and monitoring of those with HIV infection.

Children with HIV infection

The number of children in the UK with HIV infection is relatively small; however, it is known that over 300 children have died from AIDS in the UK (Molesworth and Tookey 1997). We also know that many HIV-positive women are pregnant and are unaware of their HIV status, as a result, many children may be born with HIV infection which could have been prevented (see Chapter 9). The number of children infected world-wide is frighteningly high, especially in poorer continents such as Africa.

Children may present with HIV infection in the first few months of life, often with PCP, which may be fatal in such children as the diagnosis is often only considered late. PCP in children can be prevented in the same way as in adults: by taking Septrin. Children may also present with HIV infection with indicators such as failure to thrive and severe bacterial and fungal infections. As stated in Chapter 2, children with HIV infection may also develop neurological problems causing them to 'fall off their milestones': they regress in terms of their developmental skills, that is they may stop walking and have reduced language ability and co-ordination. However, many children survive until their early teens but by this time are chronically unwell and need frequent hospital admissions. Once diagnosed, HIV-positive children may be offered anti-viral treatment. The use of anti-virals in children is less established than in adults mainly because the overall experience of such drugs in children is much more limited. Drugs are also relatively new and have really only been used extensively in adults. There are many trials using the newer drugs in children which also show promising results.

The care of children with HIV infection should ideally be carried out in specialist centres where multidisciplinary teams can be accessed and expertise is at a premium. There are numerous and complex issues around children with HIV infection which are beyond the scope of this general book. These include when to tell children the nature of their disease and the impact of HIV in a family where multiple members may be infected. However, as a rule of thumb, children are encouraged to lead a normal life. They attend nurseries and school. Who exactly needs to know about the child's HIV status is a complex issue and discussions and decisions should be made obviously in close conjunction and with the consent of other family members.

Many more children are *affected* rather than *infected* by HIV infection. As the transmission rates are relatively low, there are a larger number of children who may have HIV-positive parents than are HIV-positive themselves. This again raises complex and diverse issues beyond the scope of this book. Some include how the child will cope with increasing ill health of one or both of their parents and or siblings, the death of such family members, and who will care for the child should the parents die. Again there are no general rules but it is advisable that issues are addressed early and communication channels kept open. Each case must be dealt with on an individual basis. GPs and other community carers can call upon their experiences in other clinical circumstances. Even though they may not have cared for a family with HIV infection before they will undoubtedly have cared for families where one or more members may have a chronic debilitating illness. Many of the issues are broadly similar.

Monitoring tests

People with HIV usually attend out-patient clinics for monitoring. The most important thing to monitor is the person themselves and to enquire as to whether they have had any minor or major symptoms since the last visit. This point is often forgotten in the atmosphere of the specialist clinics where the inevitable emphasis is on the number of CD4 cells or the latest viral load figures.

CD4 count or T cell count

This is a blood test that is taken to monitor the numbers of T cells, the cells that the HIV virus infects and can be simply measured. They make up a subset of the white blood cell known as lymphocytes. These cells have a special role to play in combating viral and fungal diseases; in HIV, as T cells decrease in number, these infections are especially common. The normal range in people who are HIV-negative is 400–1000. Many people who are HIV-positive have normal T cell counts. People generally do not have major symptoms of HIV or AIDS unless their T cell count is around 300 or below, which is when they are often offered anti-viral treatment. T cells decrease as people become increasingly symptomatic from HIV and over time as the virus is able to kill more T cells. In any one day the virus may kill many T cells, however, for a time the immune system is able to replace these. It is only when the balance is turned in favour of the virus that the T cell count drops persistently.

It is important to remember that other things may influence the T cell count, which fluctuates on a day-to-day basis. Other minor infections may cause it to drop and different laboratories will give slightly different readings. People can get hooked on monitoring their T cell count and may get very upset if it drops by even a small amount. It is important that doctors clarify that it is a trend over time that is being monitored and that minor fluctuations are normal. In short, it is important to keep a balanced view when discussing T cell counts.

Viral load

A new test that has only been available since late 1996, viral load testing is also a blood test that can be performed in specialist hospitals. A large study in the United States found that viral load is what is known as a 'prognostic marker' and therefore a very important baseline and monitoring test in HIV disease (Mellors et al. 1996). The number of pieces (copies) of the HIV virus in the blood sample are measured. The range is enormous: the lowest readings will be in the hundreds, and the highest values will be over several million. This again can be confusing and requires clear explanation from the doctor. Again different laboratories may measure viral load in different ways so inevitably there will be variations in how these are expressed. As far as HIV prognosis is concerned, it is better to have a low amount of virus in the blood rather than a high amount. When someone who is not on any treatment has a high viral load this may suggest that they could progress more rapidly to symptomatic HIV and AIDS.

People with a high viral load (generally accepted to be above 100,000 copies) are often offered anti-viral treatment irrespective of their T cell count. People with a low viral load (below 10,000) may not need to start anti-viral treatment if their T cells are in the normal range. Many people fall between 10,000 and 100,000 and what exactly to do in these cases is a little less clear. However, it is generally accepted that if someone is immunosuppressed, in other words if their T cell count is 300 or below, then they should be started on anti-viral treatment.

Viral load is also a very useful measurement once someone has started on treatment. Anti-viral treatment should cause a significant fall in the viral load. This is because the drugs should cause a reduction in the viral replication, hence a fall in the viral load. In this way the continued effectiveness of treatments can be monitored and if treatments become less effective, as suggested by a persistent rise in viral load, new treatments can be tried. Some treatments are so effective that the viral load test becomes 'undetectable'. This does not mean the virus has disappeared, but is present at a very reduced level. Some confusion has arisen because of this, with some people wrongly assuming if the virus is undetectable they are not infectious to others. There is some evidence that in the era of newer treatments, more people are prepared to take risks and may become infected.

What is the link between viral loads and T cells?

Some people find it hard to piece together how CD4 counts and viral loads combine in monitoring. One way to think of it is with the following analogy. Imagine that a train station represents a person becoming unwell with AIDS and that a person is represented by a train approaching that station. The T cell count represents how far away the person is from that station and viral load test result represents the speed at which they are travelling. In other words someone with a high T cell count and a high viral load is quite a long way away from the station (in other words, from becoming ill) but is travelling quite quickly towards the station. An individual with a lower T cell count but a low viral load may be quite near the station but the viral load indicates that the train is moving more slowly towards it. The idea of anti-viral treatment in this analogy is that it effectively moves the station further away. In other words it delays the onset of major symptoms. Again viral load may be influenced by minor infections and vaccinations. Most people should have their viral load measured at least a couple of times a year and if they are thinking about starting treatment or are already on treatment then this should be done more frequently.

It is important to say, however, that viral load is a very new monitoring test and there are many questions that as yet are unanswered about it and we do not know as yet how best to use it. It is very easy for doctors and patients to get very linked into the results of this test and forget the person.

Monitoring tests are more complicated in children: their immune systems are at a different stage of development and the above information applies to adults rather than children. Interpretation of children's tests is complex and can only really be done by a paediatrician with expertise in the field.

Genetic diversity of HIV

We know that there are two distinct types of HIV virus: HIV 1 and HIV 2. As discussed in Chapter 1, HIV 1 is much more widespread. HIV 2 is largely confined to western Africa and tends to run a more indolent course than HIV 1. Several distinctive sub-types of HIV 1 have been found, and these tend to be distributed with a distinct geographic variation. These have been labelled HIV 1A, HIV 1B, HIV 1C ad infinitum. These genetic sub-types do not necessarily seem to cause different types of disease. The most common type of HIV in Europe is sub-type B. Sub-types A and D are more common in central Africa. Sub-type E is more common in Thailand and sub-type C more common in Brazil and India. The recognition of these sub-types is relevant with respect to viral load testing. This is because in a small number of people who are sub-type non-B some viral load tests may give a falsely low reading. Further complex tests need to be done to give a more accurate reading. With time, technology will improve and it is likely that this will become less of a problem.

References

Adler, M. (1993) *ABC of AIDS*, third edition, London: BMJ Publishing Group.

Johnson, M.A. and Johnstone, F.D. (eds) (1993) *HIV Infection in Women*, Edinburgh: Churchill-Livingstone.

Lipman, M.C.I., Gluck, T.A and Johnson, M.A. (1993) *A slide atlas of differential diagnosis in HIV disease*, Lancs UK/New York: Parthenon.

Mellors, J. et al. (1996) 'Prognosis in HIV-1 infection predicted by the quantity of virus in plasma', *Science*, 272: 1167–70.

Mindel, A. and Miller, R. (1996) *AIDS. A Pocket Book of Diagnosis and Management*, second edition, London: Arnold Publishing, Oxford University Press.

Molesworth, A. and Tookey, P. (1997) 'Paediatric AIDS and HIV Infection', *Communicable Disease Report Review*, 7: R132–4.

4 Meeting the Needs of People with Advancing Infection

While it is common for most clinicians, and the medical profession in general, to regard HIV infection and AIDS as a chronic condition, there is little doubt that it still has a poor prognosis. Nevertheless, this prognosis is far better than even two or three years ago and far better in comparison to the beginning of the epidemic.

This chapter highlights the needs of those patients with advancing and the advanced stages of HIV infection and AIDS. It should be seen as the first part of a 'trilogy of chapters' (the other two being Chapters 10 and 11) in which aspects of the end of life are viewed objectively, but with compassion.

This chapter provides information about the latter stages of HIV infection and AIDS and also links with the previous chapter – about the natural history of HIV infection – in this first section of the book. Furthermore it emphasises how primary care can respond to the multiple physical, psycho-social and spiritual needs of the patient. A framework is provided whereby maintenance of health, prevention, diagnosis and treatment and terminal care can be seen to be legitimate components of primary care. Finally, the principles of terminal or palliative care are described and some of the differences between home and hospice care are compared and contrasted.

One controversial topic always arising in these various debates is that of euthanasia and the related physician-assisted suicide. It is beyond the remit of this book to explore these areas comprehensively; however, the working framework for clinicians in the UK is described in order to clarify certain key points. It is the intention of the authors to provide an accurate, descriptive account of some of these issues towards the end of the chapter.

Since the epidemiology of HIV and AIDS is changing (see Chapter 3), this chapter finishes with a short piece on adoption and fostering arrangements for children from families affected by HIV infection and AIDS.

The framework for primary care

The primary care team is defined as members of a community team which provide expertise to the primary care of individuals with all types of conditions, not just HIV infection. The basic principles of effective, primary care are:

- Maintenance of good health
- Prevention of disease
- Diagnosis and treatment
- Support of patients with HIV infection
- Terminal or palliative care.

A brief description of these aspects of care is provided with a particular emphasis on HIV infection and AIDS.

Maintenance of good health

One feature of primary care in the UK, is that many people are seen on a daily basis; indeed this is one of the basic premises of many prevention programmes that are based in the community. It is estimated that two-thirds of the practice population visit the general practitioner each year and four-fifths of any population every three years. Of course, in places like London where mobility is startlingly high, these figures are less representative. Nevertheless, there is unparalleled access of primary care services to the local community.

During doctor or nurse–patient consultations, opportunistic health promotion is possible and, more specifically, sexual health promotion is now widely advocated. People who attend for vaccinations and women who consult for family planning are two examples of targeted health promotion. Some evidence shows that groups such as gay men may not see general practitioners for a variety of reasons and this can impact on HIV/AIDS education for obvious reasons. Issues such as communication and counselling skills are important in this basic aspect of care. Significant but very simple measures, such as advice about stopping smoking, may be part of an important health-promoting message which can and does benefit many people. This type of issue is an inherent part of modern-day primary care and general practice.

Prevention of disease

HIV/AIDS infection is an exemplar of how a chronic disease can be managed in the community. Factors such as its preventability, morbidity, social and psychological sequelae and overall impact on people's lives make it a condition which should rightfully have primary care input.

The wider primary care team, incorporating practice nurses, district nurses and health visitors, have a responsibility to those members of the community who 'potentially are at risk'. In addition, midwives work with well individuals on a day-to-day basis and there is increasing evidence that they are becoming more involved with HIV testing, especially in the larger conurbations where named HIV testing is being encouraged (see Chapter 9). In parts of the country where there is a high prevalence of ethnic minorities, midwives, health visitors or even 'health advocates' may have greater access to these individuals than general practitioners.

Vaccinations

In this section the traditional vaccination programmes are mentioned, for young adults (for children see Chapter 8). Many young people travel and the opportunity a consultation can provide for discussing HIV/AIDS and other sexually transmitted diseases (STDs) is enormous, so long as there is ample time (see Chapter 2).

For people with HIV infection, vaccinations are still important, though the guidelines strongly suggest that any *live* vaccines should be avoided. Thus BCG, yellow fever, oral typhoid and live, oral polio vaccines should be avoided (Salisbury and Begg 1996). Other vaccinations such as cholera, diphtheria, haemophilus influenzae type b, hepatitis A, hepatitis B, influenza, mumps/measles/rubella (MMR), meningococcal, pertussis (whooping cough), pneumococcal vaccine, poliomyelitis (by injection only), tetanus and typhoid are entirely safe. Note MMR is a live vaccine but *safe*.

An important facet of prevention is to offer hepatitis vaccinations (types A and B) to individuals who are gay (particularly men who have sex with men, or bisexuals) – there is no reason why this cannot be carried out in primary care.

Diagnosis and treatment of disease

Many HIV-related conditions can be adequately managed in general practice. General practitioners (GPs) bring to this area knowledge and skills which are often under-recognised and certainly under-used. In addition many of the factors which determine the presentation of the problem to the GP are recognised by their own doctor, for example, when a medical problem clashes with duties at work. Besides, GPs are much more aware of the certification requirements of people and will usually act as the patient's main advocate.

The very nature of HIV and AIDS means that hospital units have an important role in continuing care, and arguably this role will be increasingly important as newer medications are developed. Nevertheless, the primary role of general practice has hitherto been underestimated and yet the service is geared up to the 'diagnosis, treatment and subsequent management' of a host of conditions in a practice population. HIV infection and AIDS should be no different to any other condition in this context.

Support of patients

'Patients must be able to trust doctors with their lives and well being. To justify that trust, we as a profession have a duty to maintain a good standard of practice and care and to show respect for human life': these are the words of the General Medical Council, that is, the legislative body which monitors all doctors in the UK; furthermore, the GMC has the right to admonish or, rarely, 'strike off' doctors from the legal register.

The support of patients is the very essence of primary care and can only occur where there is familiarity with the individual, his or her informal 'family' network and their surroundings. While it has been said that many of the people affected with HIV and AIDS originated from marginal groups such as gay men or injecting drug-users, this factor should not influence how primary care services respond to the needs of particular patients.

While it has already been noted that gay men for example, tend not to use their general practitioner as widely as possible, others such as women or African women in particular use general practitioner services without problems (Madge et al. 1997).

Urban areas, especially Edinburgh, lead by example, for many general practitioners frequently treat people who inject drugs and are often HIV-positive.

Once again, people have a right to expect effective primary care services and HIV should make no difference to this; indeed many would argue that the need to have access to primary care for this diverse group is even greater.

Terminal care patients who wish to die at home

Approximately one in five patients with HIV infection and AIDS treated at a North London teaching hospital die at home (Sterling 1997). Within the community, the general practice is the ideal service to provide this type of long-term care for patients who are in the advanced stages of HIV infection and AIDS. So long as local services are familiar with the patient concerned, and their informal 'family' network, much can be done to ensure care is provided in an individually tailored way. In the field of palliative care, most interventions are geared towards enhancing the quality of life of the person with the condition. For a long time, patients with advanced HIV infection or AIDS had a very limited choice in terms of palliative care – patients were kept in hospital unnecessarily and home care could not (or would not) be arranged.

Where there is commitment from the general practitioner, the hospital services and the wider primary care team, care at home *is* possible. The obvious advantages of care at home are that care is personalised, the surroundings are familiar and there is a genuine feeling of control by the person in the last few days or weeks of their life.

Is the decision about where to die based on dogma or a genuine attempt to meet real need? While it is obvious that care in the community is the model of choice in this context, there is also some supporting evidence for this stance. For example, a Canadian study in the early 1990s surveyed the views of over 70 patients with AIDS about where they wished to die: 38 of this group opted for care at home (51 per cent). Thirty-two of the group (44 per cent) wished to die in a specialised palliative care unit, with a minority wishing to die in a hospital bed (Sterling 1997). Why should this be the case?

Two of the most powerful reasons must be control and freedom of expression. Another compelling reason must be the comfort and familiarity with the surroundings which belong to and in some way reflect the personality of the person with the disease. It has already been stated that care can be individualised. There is also something about freedom of expression at home which is not possible in an institution whether a hospice or a hospital. The disadvantage about care at home is that there must be a degree of organisation and preparation, both physically and emotionally. Support and help is mandatory and is the lynchpin of whether home care will work or not.

Paradoxically the hospital service is key in such instances because it provides important support: should a crisis arise, or an intercurrent problem (for example a chest infection that warrants aggressive therapy), an emergency admission can be arranged.

Health care workers need to realise that control – as far as the patient is concerned – is extremely important and has implications as far as 'home-visiting' is concerned. It is easy to imagine that where several care workers are visiting, perhaps on a daily basis, this can be quite intrusive for patient and carers. An awareness of this is probably all that is necessary in order to prevent the intrusion from becoming insensitive and disruptive.

Finally, because terminal care at home can be very intensive for all concerned, it is wise to think about respite care should the need arise. For example, if this period was extended to a few weeks, it may be that both patient and carers need 'a break' in which case a hospice or even brief hospital stay may be entirely appropriate.

Terminal care: patients who wish to die in a hospice

Another key service which is more common in urban areas are hospice or palliative care teams. Altogether in the United Kingdom there are over 290 hospice units comprising over 3,000 beds (Sterling 1997).

Although these general hospices provide specialist palliative care service, often as in-patient, they vary in their extent in responding to people with HIV and AIDS. It used to be the case that such services would only accept referrals if a person with HIV/AIDS had Kaposi's sarcoma, however, thankfully this ridiculous state of affairs is now outdated. In the larger cities (London, Edinburgh, Brighton), there are four special hospices which have been established in order to try and meet the needs of people with HIV infection. These hospice units provide a mixture of residential care, home-based social support and day care.

There are a number of common myths about hospices in circulation which are neither helpful nor true. First, many think that a hospice is a place to die (the same can be said about hospitals). While many people do die in hospices (because patients attending are invariably ill), hospices are now usually for short-stay, respite-type admissions. Patients are usually admitted for a short time, commonly two to three weeks, before going home again. In other words it is very common for patients to be discharged from hospices back to their own homes.

Second, and connected with the last point, many think of the hospice as being deeply religious. While many hospices have affiliations to certain religious orders, the hospice service realises the more secular state of society. People of many denominations are admitted to hospices and are discharged with their religious beliefs intact. Importantly, people of no fixed beliefs or even atheists are as welcome as anybody else in a hospice.

The most common reasons for admission to a hospice are:

- Respite care
- Symptom control/respite
- Rehabilitation
- A combination of the above.

Respite care

As implied above, caring for someone who is dying can be intensive, emotionally draining and – often underestimated – physically demanding. It is therefore wise to plan what options are available should there be a need. A hospice, where available, is an appropriate choice since one of the aims is to provide respite for the carers before the patient returns home again. In such a case the respite is useful for both patient and carers.

Symptom control and respite care

It is often a combination of factors which finally leads to an admission. For example patient and carers may be coping very well at home until a component of the 'symptom control' becomes difficult for whatever reason. Pain may suddenly become worse, or the patient may develop further symptoms (headaches, fever) and while hospital care is not appropriate a brief hospice stay may well be.

Hospices, while being institutions, are much more focused on the 'comfort and care' for the patient and also firmly believe in autonomy, in other words, that the patient's wishes are predominant. Often after a short stay and particular attention given to the troublesome symptoms which have precipitated the admission, the patient feels better and is keen to return home. Once again this break also allows the carers to recuperate for the following phase.

Rehabilitation

Rehabilitation is often a misnomer in such an instance. What is really meant is that attention to a number of aspects can result in tangible physical improvements for the patient, thus improving the patient's quality of life. For example, after a long bout of ill-health, a patient may be weak and tired and often incapable of walking unaided. This is especially common after a lengthy period of bedrest, where the patient feels trapped and claustrophobic, perhaps not having ventured out for days if not weeks. However with intensive physiotherapy or occupational therapy, a patient's strength can be harnessed to walk again. Further attention to detail, such as 'energy-saving strategies' around the house or flat, may well result in an enhanced quality of life (Cusack 1994). The same principles apply to other activities of daily living, for example washing, dressing, shaving, cleaning and cooking.

Terminal care: important elements

The important individual elements of terminal care are:

- Symptom control
- Avoidance of inappropriate therapy

- Support
- Multidisciplinary approach
- Continuity of care
- Communication.

These will be described more in detail in Chapter 9, however since it is relevant here the fundamental principles will be described.

Symptom control

There is little point in listing the vast range of 'symptoms' that an individual with advanced HIV infection and AIDS may suffer. However, a number of key 'symptom groups' will be mentioned; what is important here are the underlying principles which allow for (and ultimately provide) effective, quality terminal care.

The commonest symptom, and perhaps the worst feared by patients, is *pain*. Pain is one of the main 'symptoms' about which there is so much fear, dread and anxiety (see Chapter 9). In fact, it may be that the person (and family and/or partner) can cope with the terminal condition, but simply cannot tolerate the pain which is clearly being ineffectively controlled. In the non-AIDS population, it is said that on diagnosis of cancer, about half of all patients suffer with some type of pain and towards the end, this figure rises to almost four-fifths (OHE 1991).

In the vast majority of instances, pain can be controlled and one of the cornerstones of good, effective terminal care is the optimal management of discomfort. The secret to good pain management is to identify the cause and treat it accordingly. In terminal care, moderate doses of strong analgesics (for example morphine-type medications) can, and are, used to good effect. Unlike in the past, to witness people dying in pain is a sign that care has broken down. Pain and its control within the context of HIV infection and AIDS is fully explored in Chapter 9.

Pain control can involve other specialists, like anaesthetists. There are some rare but debilitating causes of pains which can be intractable and very difficult to relieve except with the highest doses of morphine. This may well be inappropriate since morphine also causes tiredness, somnolence and drowsiness. If a pain is localised and resistant to treatment, anaesthetists are very adept at applying their anatomical knowledge and their anaesthetic skills to suggest other ways of controlling it; it is an option worth remembering.

As in the case of patients with a non-AIDS terminal disease, other common symptoms of advanced or terminal HIV infection and AIDS include anorexia (poor appetite and weight loss), weakness, constipation, cough, nausea and vomiting, insomnia and oedema (swelling) (OHE 1991). Patients with AIDS-related complications such as pneumonia and widespread Kaposi's sarcoma (see Chapter 3) can suffer with many of these symptoms in the very advanced stages. There may well be other infections or tumours which have been resistant to other treatments.

Weight loss is a common feature which can be a problem at any time during the course of HIV infection. It is always necessary to try and identify why this is happening, and seeking the advice of the clinician is important. The causes of weight loss are multiple and sometimes can be quite complex (Summerbell 1994). It is tempting, as it is with other advanced AIDS symptoms, for the clinician to 'try another' medication; however, unless a cause is found, the patient receives a longer list of tablets, pills and potions, the majority of which do not enhance the quality of life. This is a poor state of affairs.

Weakness can be due to many reasons which will not be all stated here. Often in advancing AIDS, this is linked with poor appetite or perhaps a profound weight loss. In other instances it is the combination of these factors with an overlying depression which results in weakness. Another cause of weakness is pain; it is natural for a person with intractable pain to feel weak – the corollary is, if pain is well controlled, the person invariably feels better and stronger.

Coughing may be a problem in the pre-terminal stages, however it ought to feature less during the actual terminal stages of the disease. One of the reasons for this is that the stronger analgesics, such as morphine, have anti-cough (called antitussive) actions. One of the more common problems in very advanced disease, especially in the last few hours, is a nasty 'rattle' of the chest, which may be a harbinger of the death itself. While sometimes distressing for the patient it is always distressing for relatives and loved ones. It can be diminished rapidly with hyoscine, a medication designed to reduce the secretions ordinarily produced by the respiratory system. If immediate relief is required, an injection of hyoscine can produce relief within minutes.

Constipation is a problem that can be more than troublesome and yet is largely preventable, so long as it is anticipated. The combination of much reduced mobility, lack of appetite and side-effects of morphine often produces this irritating, yet distressing symptom. If morphine is being prescribed, it is usually good practice to also prescribe a gentle laxative. If this is already the case, then a stronger laxative is usually required, or a combination can be used. It is also important to inform the patient that, the lack of intake means their bowels will be far less active, and thus passing infrequent but soft stool is not really constipation.

Nausea and vomiting are again common problems which have a multitude of causes. As with other symptoms the cause ought to be identified and one of the most common will be adverse effects of other medications. Morphine itself is a potent stimulator of nausea, though clearly the benefits and potential side-effects ought to have been discussed beforehand. As with other symptoms clinicians can use a number of medications for nausea with good effect. Attention to diet is also important here and it may be that small, light meals are recommended, though again the advice of a dietician may pay dividends. One small point, if anti-nausea medication is given, a tablet which the patient can use sub-lingually (that is, placed under the tongue) definitely has its place.

Disfigurement can be a feature of HIV and AIDS; one of the causes, Kaposi's sarcoma (KS), has already been mentioned. The presence of cutaneous KS has been noted to be symbolic of the general stigmatisation of people with HIV and AIDS, a fate which is not only cruel but reflective of societal attitudes. This stigmatisation may be associated with feelings of guilt, depression, anxiety and ultimately with feelings of suicide. One option worth considering is the use of cosmetics. If carried out professionally, cosmetic beauticians can blank out almost all signs of KS lesions, no matter how prominent. Of course this form of 'therapy' cannot remove the lesions but it allows some release, even for a few hours, from the ever-present symbolic lesions of Kaposi's sarcoma.

Decreasing mobility also has many causes, and trying to determine which is the main reason is often very difficult. One of the biggest concerns for patients with advancing HIV infection is the combination of 'symptoms' which are cumulative. Thus, the common fear of a well person is deterioration to the point of needing much more intensive help than previously, including help with activities of daily living (such as washing and dressing). One of the most important factors here is to identify how the adjustment is being made to this new, often more serious, stage in the disease process.

It is, of course, important to note that in the advanced stages of the condition, this same combination of factors may contribute to the decreasing mobility of the affected patient. Where this is the case, the full range of the multidisciplinary team becomes involved, bringing with them their special expertise and knowledge in the various areas. It is salutary to note that at this stage it is quality of life that is the key factor, not merely quantity. How a patient judges his or her life to have sufficient quality is very much a personal, usually changeable and often unpredictable affair. However, health professionals need to know and acknowledge this, perhaps explicitly with the patient. If this is done professionally and sensitively, it allows the person to adjust relatively smoothly to the increasingly advanced stages of the condition. This approach may also allow the person – especially if they know the health professional can 'cope' with these often difficult conversations – to talk openly about impending ill-health and possibly death, and the effects it will have on others, including the family members.

Avoidance of inappropriate therapy

It is a genuine challenge for health professionals, and more importantly for the person affected, to know what is an appropriate therapy and what is inappropriate. Various arguments about what is and is not appropriate ultimately depend on whose perspective is being taken; in other words is it the patient's view, the relative's, the general practitioner's, the specialist or even someone else? Of course, where a consensus is reached, and everyone agrees, decisions become straightforward.

Whether 'active' treatments ought to be given in terminal care or whether total parenteral nutrition ought to be commenced in patients with AIDS are questions not easily resolved. Where treatments are plainly futile the crucial question is where to 'draw the line', though what constitutes futile will always be debated.

Support

One reason why primary care can respond to the needs of patients with advancing disease is that, for much of this time, patients will be at home anyway. The support of the HIV and AIDS-affected patient by members of the primary care team, including the GP, is a potentially vital aspect of this care. This aspect is no different in the advancing stages as it was earlier, indeed arguably it is more important in the latter stages.

One of the most difficult challenges for health care workers is to care for a patient who appears to be in persistent or relentless pain. This scenario often requires the active collaboration of health, social and voluntary agencies to try and diminish the suffering of the patient. It is easily forgotten, especially in such a secular society as the UK, that a religious leader or representative could well help here more than any medical clinician. Anxiety, guilt and dread can be the indirect cause of this overall pain and religious input may well be very helpful in such circumstances.

Multidisciplinary approach

It should be abundantly clear that to provide good, effective, sensitive care to people with advanced HIV infection or AIDS often requires the help, support and skills of a number of professions (Cusack and Singh 1994). The traditional role of the *general practitioner (GP)* as a community doctor is sustained on account of several nursing specialities who can complement this care in people's homes. It is not without coincidence that HIV/AIDS has been noted to be the exemplar of a chronic condition. Thus, nursing input may consist of *palliative nurse specialists, MacMillan nurses, district nurses*, and special *liaison HIV/AIDS nurses* who have specialist knowledge and skills in this area.

A *physiotherapist* may also be very useful in this regard though their role extends further than one which is solely concerned with mobility. Physiotherapists have specialist knowledge in respiratory conditions and neurological problems, especially where these impinge upon a person's ability to look after themselves (McClure 1994). Of course one dimension of this may be mobility.

For other mobility needs an *occupational therapist (OT)* may be very useful; and often in such an example the roles of the occupational therapist and the physiotherapist overlap. The former has special skills in ensuring the vital 'activities of daily living' can be carried out in a safe and secure way. An effective occupational therapist may provide ideas about how a person's home can be adapted including the bathroom, kitchen or bedroom (Cusack 1994). Because a detailed OT assessment can take a few hours (longer if done in the person's home), the occupational therapist has a particularly good idea of the mental state of the person. Issues such as the person's memory, overall motivation, levels of anxiety or even depression may be firmly gauged by the OT on such a visit. The usefulness of this information for the clinicians should never be underestimated and may, in the long run, help to plan services for the person affected.

Another useful therapist is the *dietician* whose role in caring for a person with HIV or AIDS can be very useful, especially where symptoms related to the digestive system are common (Summerbell 1994). Specialist HIV therapists are harder to access out of the large cities, but a generic therapist along these lines may have ideas and experience of their own.

For people who require ongoing help, support in the form of a generic *social worker* is invaluable. Their professional role is a combination of health and social advice, welfare rights, counsellor and personal friend and no less valued for it (Bairstow 1994). Although their roles are forever changing, they are often in the unenviable position whereby too little or too much intervention attracts criticism which is nearly always destructive. They are often called upon to perform in the most trying of circumstances with the most challenging of patients in an environment where resources are inevitably constrained.

One clinician often forgotten but of vital importance is the *dentist*. The principles which determine the need for a dentist are no different because a person is HIV-positive. It has been estimated that about a third of people stop attending their dentist on finding out about their status (Croser et al. 1994), either because they fear refusal, have concerns about confidentiality or harbour genuine fears about infecting others. As is the case with general practitioners, some people will continue to attend without informing the dentist about their status, often for similar reasons.

A person with chronic HIV infection requires dental surveillance and treatment just as much as any other person with a serious medical condition (see Chapter 3). Thus, freedom from pain, restored function and aesthetic considerations are critical in the context of a person's dental health. Dental treatment ought to be planned with the middle to long term in mind, especially taking into account the much better prognosis for a person with HIV nowadays.

As in other conditions, the emphasis on acute care and prevention – a facet of care which is just as relevant in dentistry as in general medicine – is entirely appropriate. Indeed HIV and AIDS commonly impacts on the teeth and on the mouth in general, often causing much pain and distress. It is also not uncommon to find that people tolerate persistent mouth or dental pain even though it is severe enough to reduce markedly their daily intake of food. The full range of infections – be they fungal, viral or bacterial – and neoplasms (tumours) can affect both the gums and the teeth, hence the need for monitoring and good dental care. In the mouth itself, there are several causes of ulceration to the gums which are associated with chronic HIV infection, many of which are eminently treatable. Finally how dental services are accessed will depend on the service available. In larger cities, specialised HIV clinics have been established for this group of people and it is imperative that the traditional dentist can liaise with these clinics accordingly. In other places, specialised dental clinics are attached to GU clinics, dedicated HIV/AIDS clinics or even special hospital departments.

Continuity of care

Continuity of care is often, from the health professional's point of view, difficult to provide. For the person living with HIV or AIDS, continuity is as vital a component of care as, for example, follow-up hospital appointments or receiving the right medication. General practitioners have felt that one of their particular strengths has been 'continuity of care', though, as has been stated before, certain people with HIV/AIDS have not been in a position to experience this in any meaningful way. This is especially so in larger urban areas where both patient turnover, and the nature of inner-city practice act as barriers to overall continuity of care. Where it works, this type of continuity can work very well and the patient can benefit tangibly from a service which is local, available and accessible.

Communication

As can be gleaned from the above sections, these components of care, if they are to work well, require forethought, planning, attention to detail and, probably above all, communication between all members of the team. At this point it is necessary to state that communication with and for the person affected by HIV or AIDS is an absolute must. The days of medical paternalism – where doctors or health professionals made decisions for the patient (often without them even knowing about it!) – are now fast receding. It is wise at this juncture to emphasise the basic care structure in the UK, these being the hospital and community sectors of care. Thus, usually, most people – whatever their condition – will be at home. If the person affected becomes ill or develops worrying symptoms then either the general practitioner can attempt to treat this in the community (see Chapter 6) or a referral can be made to the hospital (see Chapter 7), either as an emergency or via an out-patient department. One of the problems up to now in the HIV/AIDS field has been an underemphasis on care in the community for people with HIV. Reasons for this are often complex and muddled by several other factors. It is also highly dependent on the area of focus, for example in some cities in Scotland, general practitioners have always played a central role in the care of people with HIV infection.

When a person with HIV sees a hospital physician, the specialist should always communicate with the general practitioner as is the case in many other conditions. The problem with HIV treatment in some areas in the UK is that the organisation of core services is based upon the genito-urinary clinic (sometimes called the sexually transmitted disease (STD) service). In this case the hospital clinic may be very reluctant to communicate with the GP because of a heightened notion of confidentiality.

Because of the nature of STD clinics, there is a law which states no information can be passed on to any agency without the expressed desire of the person concerned. Of course this is what should happen anyway in any other field of medicine and clinical practice, except, that in STD clinics it is covered by statute. Where does this leave the person affected by HIV or AIDS?

Sometimes it leaves them without the support and help from their community doctor. Sometimes it will make no difference whatsoever, because, to the credit of the hospital clinics, the care received is absolutely exemplary. Nevertheless, where this communication has broken down between hospital and GP, it leaves the patient quite vulnerable since the GP will not have the benefit of the available information. A number of research papers have explored this topic to the full and it is beyond the remit of this chapter to explore this further. Nevertheless, the bottom line of these arguments are that for effective care to take place, communication is mandatory.

Euthanasia

Euthanasia and other related subjects are very emotive; however, there are specific and fairly rigorous guidelines laid down by, for example the General Medical Council. Euthanasia has been described as 'the compassion-motivated, deliberate, rapid, and painless termination of life of someone afflicted with an incurable and progressive disease' (Boyd et al. 1997). In other words it is the conscious ending of a person's life on account of their wishes and usually carried out by a clinician, most frequently a doctor.

The problem with this doctor-assisted process (whether euthanasia or suicide) is that it is not officially part of the doctor's role according to the General Medical Council (GMC). Indeed their stance along with that of the British Medical Association is that a doctor ought to 'prevent suffering, relieve suffering and heal the sick'. Euthanasia is therefore not part of this role and many doctors as well as lay people are concerned that one of the central tenets of medical ethics, that of 'first do no harm', will have been violated. Hence quite simply euthanasia should not be allowed.

So where does that leave the present thinking about euthanasia? Here a number of problems remain unclear and thus unresolved. While officially euthanasia is not allowed, certain surveys and questionnaires involving GPs and others admit that they have terminated the life of patients whose suffering was thought to be unbearable. In some countries, the most famous being The Netherlands, euthanasia is 'allowed', although even there it is technically still a criminal act. Because of this ambiguity, doctors can find the system very stressful; this will be discussed below.

Ethical arguments about euthanasia

One reason why dilemmas surround euthanasia is that it somehow contravenes the ordinary person's expectations about a doctor's central role. In other words, most people do not expect doctors to wilfully end life. As a result many ethicists argue that once doctors are allowed to do this, for example in cases of extreme suffering, then the sanctity of the doctor's role will never be the same again. Furthermore, one of the most basic ethical guides for doctors is that they 'should first do no harm'. Evidently euthanasia does not stand up to this first basic rule of medical ethics. Of course, taken from the patient's perspective, this may seem inflexibly unreasonable.

A second argument against euthanasia is that it somehow detracts from the relatively rapid rise in terminal or palliative care expertise that the UK has witnessed over the last 20 to 30 years. This expertise (and the associated movement in general), which was initiated by Dame Cicely Saunders, has continued to flourish in hospices, academic units, hospitals and community units. There are now over 3,000 beds for patients with a terminal condition in almost 300 hospice units throughout the UK, including four specialist HIV/AIDS units. Nevertheless, the majority of people who die, irrespective of disease process, die in a hospital. The argument is that this effort will therefore be wasted if euthanasia is resorted to by patients with a terminal condition.

Finally, and importantly especially where relatives or carers are concerned, many people, perhaps those who are particularly elderly may feel the pressure of remaining alive and request 'out of a sense of duty' that euthanasia be carried out.

The arguments *for* euthanasia are equally powerful. Many people argue that to prolong life, irrespective of the condition or the extent of suffering is tantamount to prolonging the suffering of both patients and relatives or carers. People invoke the cry of 'they would not inflict that upon a stray dog'. This is easily understandable in some circumstances, especially if the patient is already very ill, for example with a rapidly progressive condition whose only course is 'downhill' and for which medicine cannot offer anything but palliation.

Another compelling reason why euthanasia can be justified is that a patient's autonomy taken to its logical conclusion would allow this to occur. Of course many would argue that a person wishing to die cannot be 'rational', in which case the argument would be lost. It is perhaps useful to describe the situation in Holland where these types of cases have brought the argument sharply into focus.

Euthanasia in The Netherlands

Many people cite the case of The Netherlands where apparently euthanasia is allowed. However, the position in The Netherlands is far from clear and this ambiguity in many ways is unhelpful.

First, there are a number of guidelines that doctors *must follow* or they risk conviction in cases of euthanasia or assisted suicide (this latter term refers to something that may be preferable for doctors, but the outcome may be less certain). Euthanasia can only be carried out following the repeatedly expressed wishes of an individual, which are then formalised in a document and witnessed. It must be agreed that the patient has less than six months to live and be suffering with a condition that results in 'hopelessness with permanent and unbearable suffering'. Another independent doctor must be part of this process. Finally, once euthanasia has taken place, the doctor – either specialist or general practitioner – must report this 'unnatural death' to the equivalent of the coroner. An agreement between the various Dutch medical and legal authorities ensures that a doctor who follows this protocol will not be taken to court, however there are now many cases where this has not been followed. This is why the practice is very stressful for doctors and from the preceding description it is clear that the doctor will have performed a criminal act (Churchill and King 1997). A recent case of a doctor who did not follow this agreed schedule resulted in him being charged with murder (Sheldon 1997).

Of course this procedure is not without its problems and certainly doctors who do not wish to offer 'this type of service' are encouraged to refer the patient to someone who would be open to such discussions. Another problem is no one is really sure how common the request is, nor how many times the set procedures are not followed, even though this entails considerable risk to the doctors. It is clear that balancing the legal requirement to report all such cases with the needs of the Dutch population in terms of regulation and monitoring abuse is genuinely difficult.

Once again, this system is unique to The Netherlands: euthanasia is not allowed in the UK. It seems fairly obvious now that such acts take place, however, any clinician risks their livelihood if it was revealed that they had taken part in such an act. The General Medical Council for doctors would certainly not tolerate such behaviour. In addition, many would argue, as stated above, that it is ultimately a failure of the terminal care management of a patient for a person to request euthanasia. Thus treatment of underlying symptoms and a review of a patient's psycho-emotional state are the necessary requirements for such an individual.

Anticipating future needs

One of the main points to arise from this book is that adjustment to HIV infection and AIDS is often the key to a quality of life that is acceptable and tolerable. A key question in the lives of people with HIV infection, particularly for women though not exclusively so, is what will happen to the children? Of course these questions are more focused in families in which more than one member is already HIV-positive (see case histories in Chapter 9).

When working with people with advancing HIV infection, part of the adjustment process is to ensure that legal and emotional guardians are duly appointed. The legalities of such a circumstance are straightforward, although the practicalities are always less so (Hogg 1996).

Guardianship

Many of the following points arise directly from the Children's Act of 1989. The partner of a woman, whether still married or in the case of legal separation, is responsible for a child if the mother was to die. If no other parent exists the welfare of the child falls into the care of the local authority. In order to ensure guardianship formal arrangements can be made as in a will. A friend or relative can take care of children, but only if there is no partner, or, for example the father has not made plans to take legal responsibility as parent. More than one person can be appointed as guardian and this is normally valid until the child reaches 18 years of age. There is no direct financial help, although the person(s) may be entitled to a special but small Guardians' Allowance from the state.

Permanent arrangements for children

Foster care or adoption is an option worth considering where there is no close relative or appropriate friend willing to take on what will be quite a responsibility. Fostering is an arrangement whereby the local authority pays for the child to be cared for over a short period; nevertheless both the child and the parent ought to be involved in this process. As time goes on, it may be that more and more parenting is carried out by the foster parents than the 'real' parents. Though this is tragic, at least the parents know the child or children are being capably cared for.

   Adoption is the more formal, permanent solution whereby legal transfer of the child is made to the new family. Although more suitable for younger children, where security is a premium, the older child may justify a prolonged long-term fostering arrangement. It is the task of specialist social workers to try and organise this in the most sensitive and competent way possible.

Box 4.1   Questions to think about when choosing a legal guardian

- How does the proposed guardian feel about the responsibility?
- How does the child feel about this arrangement?
- How has the guardian brought up their children?
- Would the child fit into this new family?
- Would you prefer one or more guardians?
- Will the guardian keep in touch with the 'family'?
- Will the guardian respect family traditions?

This is a relatively specialised area and further information can be obtained from:

The British Agencies for Adoption and Fostering
11, Southwark Street,
London SE1 1RQ
Phone: 0171 407 8800

Scottish Adoption Association
2, Commercial Street,
Leith,
Edinburgh EH6 6JA
Phone: 0131 553 5060

Summary

One reason why general practice is so successful is that it provides care which is accessible, available, flexible and, by and large, free at the point of delivery. An important component of this is that it should be continuous and user-friendly, especially for people who hitherto have suffered their fair share of stigma and rejection.

In the special case of palliative care the patient with AIDS can be maintained in comfort and in familiar surroundings. The patient's choice and control are the central features in this circumstance. For the patient with HIV infection or AIDS, the benefits of this local service working alongside the specialist care centres can pay dividends in many different ways.

Ultimately it is symptom control – taking the whole patient into account – and the will to communicate which tangibly determines how effective this care will be. Doctors, nurses and the whole team ought to be orchestrated by the needs of the patient. In advancing HIV infection or AIDS, the patient often cannot do this alone, or needs to be accompanied by a partner, close friend or family member. The process may be slower but no less intense for those concerned.

In cases where serious decisions need to be made, or where such decisions can be anticipated, pre-planning with the production of an advanced directive or a living will may be the answer (see Chapter 10 for details). The *real* advocate for the patient – and this is not necessarily the 'next-of-kin' – ought to be identified earlier rather than later. Often their role will be immensely helpful when major decisions need to be made in the last few hours or days of life.

One of these 'major' decisions is who will look after the children and this chapter provides basic information on the options for adoption and fostering. Clearly this type of anticipatory care is all the more sad but necessary. Good, effective, personally tailored care requires just this anticipation in order to provide a judicious, balanced attention to those affected by HIV infection.

References

Bairstow, S. (1994) 'The Social Worker's Role' in Cusack, L. and Singh, S. (eds) *HIV & AIDS Care: Practical approaches*, London: Chapman & Hall.
Boyd, K.M., Higgs, R. and Pinching, A.J. (1997) *The New Dictionary of Medical Ethics*, London: BMJ Publishing Group.
Churchill, L.R. and King, N.M.P. (1997) 'Physician assisted suicide, euthanasia, or withdrawal of treatment', editorial, *British Medical Journal*, 315: 137–8.
Croser, D., Erridge, P. and Robinson, P. (1994) *HIV and Dentistry – A guide to dental treatment for patients with HIV and AIDS*, BDA Occasional Paper, Issue 4, November.
Cusack, L. (1994) 'The role of the Occupational Therapist' in Cusack, L. and Singh, S. (eds) *HIV & AIDS Care: Practical approaches*, London: Chapman & Hall.
Cusack, L. and Singh, S. (1994) *HIV & AIDS Care: Practical approaches*, London: Chapman & Hall.
General Medical Council (GMC) (1995) *Duties of a doctor*, Guidance from the GMC, London: GMC.
Hogg, C. (1996) *Living Positively: A guide for parents and carers*, London: National Children's Bureau.
Madge, S., Olaitan, A., Morcroft, A., Phillips, A.N. and Johnson, M.A. (1997) 'Access to medical care one year prior to diagnosis in one hundred HIV positive women', *Family Practice*, 14: 255–7.
McClure, J. (1994), 'The Role of the Physiotherapist' in Cusack, L. and Singh, S. (eds) *HIV & AIDS Care: Practical approaches*, London: Chapman & Hall.
OHE (Office of Health Economics) (1991) *Dying with dignity*, No. 97 in a series of reports about health problems, London: OHE.
Salisbury, D.M. and Begg, N.T. (eds) (1996) *Immunisation against infectious disease*, London: Department of Health.
Sheldon, T. (1997) 'Dutch GP in euthanasia will not go to prison', *British Medical Journal*, 314: 1148.
Sterling, C. (1997), '"Where to die": Aspects of shared care and responsibility', *Lecture at Royal College of Physicians/Royal College of GPs*, 9 Oct. 1997.
Summerbell, C. (1994) 'Nutrition in HIV disease' in Cusack, L. and Singh, S. (eds) *HIV & AIDS Care: Practical approaches*, London: Chapman & Hall.

5   Mental Health and HIV

HIV infection not only impacts on physical health but also can affect an individual's mental health and psychological well-being. This may occur in several ways.

HIV infection when first diagnosed can sometimes precipitate severe mental illness such as depression or psychosis, though this happens rarely. Lay people sometimes call this a 'nervous breakdown'. However, more often it causes mild symptoms that may or may not need treatment other than support. It is important to remember that the impact of an HIV diagnosis would naturally raise levels of anxiety therefore it is not surprising that many people at one time or another may have symptoms of mild depression.

Some people who have HIV infection have a pre-existing diagnosis or vulnerability to mental health disorders. In other words they may already have had an episode of depression, an abnormal personality or be diagnosed as schizophrenic. HIV may worsen these problems.

HIV itself can cause abnormalities in the brain and this might cause a change in personality. For example, HIV can cause a dementia. Other complications such as toxoplasmosis can start off with changes in personality. Usually this occurs in people who are unwell with advanced HIV disease and who have low CD4 counts.

In other ways HIV can lead to changes in mental health. For example, drugs prescribed by doctors and some non-prescribed drugs that people take may cause changes in personality and behaviour.

It is not always easy to work out exactly what is the cause for changes in mental health. In fact it can be quite complicated and a challenge for all concerned including the person affected. Therefore, doctors are often cautious and will exclude 'medically' treatable causes first. This means that patients can be investigated quite intensively with brain scans and other tests before a diagnosis of mental illness is made. HIV specialist doctors may ask for help from other specialists to clarify the situation such as neurologists and psychiatrists (see Chapter 6).

Maintaining good mental health

There are some simple ways that someone who has HIV infection can keep their mental health in a good state. Some ideas are listed below.

- Most people find a balance and integrate their HIV diagnosis into their life. This is better than either denying that there is a problem at all or allowing HIV to take over. However, finding a balance can be difficult and some people find that operating at the extremes is what works best for them.
- For most people it is better to keep busy; ideally in a job that they find motivating. This provides a structure to their time and an income; however, some people choose not to work or cannot find work. Some people may find that they've given up work perhaps too soon and boredom has taken over, which may increase the probability of reflecting and ruminating about HIV.
- A good network of close friends or family who are supportive, or ideally a combination of the two, is highly valuable. People can still be supportive in various ways even if they may not know about the HIV diagnosis.
- Moderation in terms of alcohol, cigarettes and other drugs is preferable, although quite often once someone is depressed they can easily get into a vicious circle of using more drinks and drugs that will worsen their depression and physical health. Alcohol is a depressant and cannabis, for example, can de-motivate people. Cigarettes may cause chest problems, which are more common with HIV anyway. Other drugs which may cause initial euphoria, such as amphetamines or 'ecstasy', are also linked to symptoms of depression with continued use.
- Regular physical exercise is good for an individual's mental health, as well as being good for physical health. Exercise can also reduce stress, provide a social role and can aid relaxation.
- A good diet, avoiding stress and finding one's own personal mechanism for coping with stress is beneficial, for example, pursuing hobbies and taking regular holidays.
- Finally if things are not going well then it is always best to ask for help. There is a considerable range of support and help that can be offered to people with HIV who are experiencing problems with their mental health.

The above list is an *aide-mémoire* of 'things a person can do to help themselves' and hence generalisations appear with regularity. For any one person it is very difficult to 'prescribe' how best to keep one's mental health in top form. Some of the points made above also apply to those caring for people with HIV in a professional capacity. It is widely acknowledged that doctors in particular are not as good as they could be at looking after their own mental health. For this reason we have included material on 'burnout' and maintaining boundaries at the end of this chapter. In the rest of the chapter we will address some specific times and situations when the mental health of those with HIV may be affected.

At HIV diagnosis

When someone is told that they are HIV-positive, they may be quite shocked. Some people go into a period of denial where they do not believe the result and it may take several weeks or months to adjust to this new situation. At HIV diagnosis some people become depressed and occasionally suicidal. However, there are various factors that may lessen the risk of depression and therefore suicide after diagnosis.

Spending some time discussing specific issues around HIV testing before taking the test is highly advisable. Discussion usually focuses particularly on how the person might cope with a positive result, whom they would tell and what would be their main concern; this chance to talk may lessen the impact when given a positive result (see Chapter 2). Very occasionally some people have an HIV test without their consent or without fully realising the implications of doing so. Sometimes this means that getting the result is a great shock and more time may be needed in such circumstances.

Existing support networks are very important at the time of diagnosis. Most people choose to tell at least one or two close friends or family members; some people choose not to tell anyone and this may increase their stress. However, they would all be offered support by the hospital services, general practitioner (GP) or other specialist services. Others are entirely open about their HIV status. Discussing the informal social network of the person is quite important; for example the patient may *want* someone to know while they also feel others *ought* to be told about their HIV diagnosis. These are significant elements of the pre-test discussion.

Another important factor in pre-test assessment for health care workers is that they should assess an individual's pre-existing personality. Someone who has a previous history of depression may be at greater risk when taking an HIV test and need extra support at time of giving the result.

Some people who test for HIV are very well prepared for an HIV-positive result. They may have been considering testing for a long time and, often, strangely, the confirmation of their fears can relieve some of their anxiety.

For some patients the time around HIV diagnosis can be particularly difficult and they may experience what is known as 'anniversary reactions' when the date of diagnosis is reached in future years.

The two short case histories below exemplify how in different situations people cope with the new diagnosis of HIV infection.

Case history: CP

CP is a 24-year-old man. He was working as a carer for people with HIV infection. He had a partner, JL, who had died six months previously from AIDS. CP himself had never taken an HIV test although he knew at the beginning of his relationship with JL that there were some sexual risks. Some time after JL's death he felt it was time to establish his own HIV status and he went for a test. When given his positive result he was not entirely shocked. He felt a certain element of relief as he could now plan how he might manage his future and he had been anxious not knowing his HIV status.

He has been supported by hospital and community services, however, he has had a very difficult year. After several months the impact of the loss of his partner and his new HIV diagnosis 'really seemed to hit him'. He became depressed and his work was becoming a major issue. Since his job was caring for people with HIV infection, there seemed no escape from his predicament. He found he had to stop work. At the same time, unfortunately, his housemates sold their house and he had to move.

Being unemployed he had to seek help financially from state benefits, which is stressful in itself, as well as rehouse himself. He was given help with this. His two closest friends who moved out of the house, moved out of London and his most immediate natural support networks were lost.

During this time he had decided to tell his mother his diagnosis. He anticipated that his mother would be supportive but unfortunately this proved not to be the case. Hence the recent loss of his partner, job, house and close friends compounded the impact of his HIV diagnosis. This meant that CP had an extremely difficult year, needing much support from hospital and community services. During this whole time CP's physical health was good. His immunological results were very satisfactory but this seemed to offer him very little comfort and only add to his uncertainty.

Case history: MC

MC is a 38-year-old bisexual man who had been a drug user back in his home town in the former Yugoslavia. He had been thinking about having an HIV test for many years. He had known several friends who had died from AIDS and knew that he had put himself at risk not only sexually but also through shared needle use. He discussed testing for HIV on several occasions with his GP, and also with a dermatologist to whom he was referred by his GP because of increasing skin problems. These were thought to be HIV-related.

After many months of consideration he went for an HIV test and on receiving the positive result, again, was not at all surprised. He attended his appointment for the test with a friend, who was also with him when he received his positive result. His major concerns were how advanced the infection was and what his immune results showed. He proved to have very advanced disease and needed to start on combination anti-viral therapy and Septrin (Co-trimoxazole) as pneumocystis carinii pneumonia (PCP) prophylaxis over the next few visits.

The most difficult thing for MC to cope with was not his HIV diagnosis, but the immunological results. His first CD4 count came back as 4 and his viral-load was 254,000. However, he needed less support than the previous patient. He had a good network of friends who all knew that he was considering having an HIV test and were all supportive after he had received his positive result. He also had stable employment with which he continued. This provided him with a structure for his time and also an income. Work proved to be somewhat of a distraction in terms of side-effects when he started on his combination anti-viral treatment. He needed far less input from hospital and community services than the previous patient although his immune results were much worse.

Depression

Depression is a term used by the lay public very frequently. For doctors, depression that is severe enough to warrant interventions, either medical treatments or counselling, usually presents with some of the following symptoms:

- Loss of appetite

- Loss of weight
- Inability to sleep – either not being able to get to sleep or waking up early in the morning
- Mood changes – more typically worse in the morning
- Feeling low in energy and feeling tired all the time
- Fearfulness
- Irritability
- A loss of sexual drive
- Negative feelings about other people
- Impaired ability to concentrate, for example, while trying to read a book or watch a film
- Feelings of low self-esteem and worthlessness
- Loss of interest in their personal appearance and their personal hygiene.

Some people who are depressed may contemplate suicide – this may be in a rather vague and abstract way, perhaps on the basis that 'not being here' may have its advantages. Others may have made more fixed plans such as thinking out how they might end their life, storing tablets up to do this, writing letters to loved ones and this represents a more serious risk of suicide. Sometimes it may be difficult for either a doctor or a patient to easily recognise depression. Some people do not want to tell anyone quite how bad they are feeling. However, once a diagnosis has been reached, discussing various treatment options with the patient is the next stage.

There are drugs that are very effective in treating depression. Many people have heard of Prozac, which is sometimes used. Other drugs include Amytriptyline and Dothiepin, which are used especially if someone is having problems sleeping. All anti-depressants have side-effects and it is wise to discuss these before starting on a course of treatment. Anti-depressants in the same group as Prozac may work within a few days; others take a few weeks. It is advisable to stay on a course of treatment for several months.

Other options for treatment such as regular individual sessions with a counsellor can be of benefit, although actual proof that it is absolutely advantageous is still a matter of debate. Sometimes, group work can be helpful. Other types of therapy include cognitive therapy that focuses much more on 'the here and now' and altering patterns of established behaviour.

Mild depression can be easily managed by a general practitioner. GPs are very experienced in managing depression in the community. If depression is very severe, psychiatric help may be sought and follow-up with community psychiatric nurses can be helpful. Only in severe cases is it necessary to admit someone to hospital with depression.

Some people find that alternative or complementary therapies can be helpful when they are feeling depressed.

Psychotic illness

This is a more extreme form of mental illness, when a person loses touch with reality. The symptoms may, however, be only intermittent making it difficult to diagnose. However, some symptoms that a person may present include extreme withdrawal, bizarre ideas and strange behaviour. People may have very fixed and yet very odd ideas that they firmly believe despite evidence to the contrary. These are called *delusions*, for example, someone may believe they are being poisoned or talked about by others. They might also experience hearing voices. These are called *auditory hallucinations*. They may also experience transfers of energy from objects to people. The causes of such extreme symptoms may be:

- Occasionally *HIV* itself can cause a psychosis.
- *Severe depression* may lead to a psychotic illness.
- A person who has pre-existing *schizophrenia* can suffer with episodes of psychosis.
- *Drugs* such as cannabis and ecstasy may sometimes lead to psychotic illnesses.
- Rarely drugs *prescribed* by doctors can cause a psychotic illness, for example very high doses of steroid medication.

Because of the severity of the symptoms when someone is psychotic, often expert psychiatric help is warranted and admission to hospital is necessary. If this is against the individual's wish, the Mental Health Act can be instigated: a doctor and a social worker can 'commit' someone to hospital for a period of time. This period of time is dependent on the section of the Mental Health Act (1983) which has been applied for. The Act contains a number of sections for both assessment and treatment of a mental condition and is only invoked in serious cases. This is relatively rare and only used in extreme cases as often someone can be persuaded to come into hospital voluntarily. Despite reports to the contrary, doctors and social workers do not like to admit people to hospital involuntarily, and a number of safeguards are in place to ensure this is not abused. If however someone is deemed 'a danger to themselves or others', then admission to hospital is sought for obvious reasons.

Treatments for psychotic illness are largely through drug therapies, often injections, and follow-up once someone has improved is usually needed via community psychiatric nurses. Specialist support groups with supervision also exist in the community and people can get advice and support from advice groups such as MIND or SANE (see Useful Addresses).

AIDS dementia

HIV-associated dementia was first described in 1986. HIV can cause brain impairment which may be, in some cases, a serious dementia. Symptoms can be much milder in many people with, for example, minimal memory loss that does not need any specific treatment other than practical measures such as making lists. However people with progressive dementia need an enormous amount of input in terms of home care services and may ultimately need carers who provide support for them 24 hours a day. Unfortunately, people with rapidly progressive HIV dementia often only live for six months to a year after the diagnosis is made. AZT and other anti-virals may slow down the progression of the disease itself but unfortunately only rarely are dramatic improvements seen.

HIV dementia is a global dementia, in other words this means that it causes changes in someone's behaviour, thought processes and subsequently, physical performance. It is most common in people who have advanced HIV infection although in some cases it can occur in people who have previously been quite well. What actually causes HIV dementia is unclear. It does seem to be a direct effect of the HIV virus on the brain and spinal cord, rather than an infection due to a secondary opportunistic organism. With the increased use of AZT and other combination therapies in recent years, there has been a reduction in the proportion of patients with serious AIDS-related dementia when compared to the late 1980s. There is some concern that some of the newer anti-virals, which do not seemingly penetrate the nervous system to the same degree as AZT, may mean that there will be an increase in AIDS dementia in the future.

Children with HIV infection may develop a syndrome related to neurological damage caused by HIV where they 'fall off their milestones': their development in terms of mobility (walking, crawling and so on) and other skills such as fine movements and language do not develop normally and, indeed, start to recede. This syndrome is not uncommon in children with HIV infection and there is evidence that AZT is, again, very useful in halting the progression of such neurological disease.

As previously stated, other AIDS-related illness can present with altered behaviour and changes in someone's mental state (Harrison and McArthur 1995). These infections include PML, toxoplasmosis and lymphomas (see Chapter 3). These are all serious but treatable to a different extent and are diagnosed by different investigations. They are generally confined to people who have advanced HIV disease and very low CD4 counts. People who have PML or lymphomas in the brain often have a very poor outlook on the whole and 'quality of life' becomes the predominant issue for those affected.

Sexual dysfunction

Many people with HIV will complain, at one time or another, of altered sexual function. This in itself is extremely common in the general population but is often under-reported. The impact of an HIV diagnosis, itself a sexually transmitted disease, will often bring sexual concerns to the fore. The impact of the diagnosis itself is frequently enough to cause a transient loss in libido (sex drive). Often people newly diagnosed with HIV infection say they will 'never have sex again'. It is important to reassure them that libido does return. Due to the transmissible nature of HIV, dialogue regarding sexual matters must occur to minimise the risk of the person getting other sexually transmitted diseases and also passing on HIV to others.

Sexual concerns are something that many people feel embarrassed to discuss and it is often assumed, wrongly, that these concerns are the responsibility of 'other' health care professionals. All health care workers may assume that everyone else is discussing sexual concerns with the patient when, in fact, nobody is. No assumption should be made as to whether or not someone is sexually active. It is only by asking direct questions in a tactful and sensitive way that the necessary information can be elicited and any problems discussed and solutions suggested. Other causes for loss in libido should be considered in someone with HIV. It may be a symptom of depression. Some prescribed drugs can cause impotence in men and loss of libido in women. Sexual dysfunction may also be caused by other coexisting illnesses such as diabetes. As HIV can often cause damage to the nervous system, this may manifest itself as impotence.

There are often special clinics that people can be referred to if they have persistent sexual problems. These can be extremely helpful in excluding a physical cause for sexual problems and also offering a range of treatments to improve their sex life.

Counselling

Counselling is rather a vague term and somewhat 'fashionable' in recent times. Doctors, as a part of their consultation, perform counselling, as do other health care workers. Counselling could be defined as a 'discussion by which concerns are raised and addressed, psychological health is assessed and decisions are facilitated within a supportive environment' (Mindel and Miller 1996.) This does not necessarily mean that you have to 'like' your counsellor or that you should see them as a friend. Counselling often necessarily addresses difficult subjects and therefore may make people feel worse initially as problems are raised before solutions can be identified and acted upon.

In the context of HIV infection many patients seek sessions of counselling either within the hospital or in the voluntary sector or GPs surgeries. These may be a fixed number of sessions where specific problems are identified and sessions are quite focused. It is unusual for these to go on for more than an hour. Usually counselling sessions occur in a one-to-one situation although couple counselling can be very productive especially when people are experiencing relationship problems. Group counselling can also be effective, for example, for people who have recently discovered their HIV status. Here those affected can get support from others in similar situations. Carers too can gain support from group work.

Counselling can continue throughout HIV disease (Miller and Madge 1996). Counselling is however a word that is subject to fashions in medicine. If counselling means information-sharing and allowing an individual with HIV to make decisions about their life, then clearly much of this is an ever-continuing process. Most people have a discussion about HIV testing before the HIV test is performed and will be 'counselled' following their HIV-positive result.

When someone is well with minimal symptoms from their HIV, counselling can be helpful to enable people to continue with their life in terms of work and relationships. Counselling can help people to disclose their diagnosis to others. Concerns for the future can be addressed at this time and decisions, such as family planning, children, practising safer sex, are frequently raised. Starting on treatment is a big step and may raise issues such as who else knows the diagnosis, changing lifestyle, the need to disclose diagnosis. Counselling can again help some people through this stage.

When people become more ill with symptoms of HIV infection or AIDS itself, counselling can be helpful as this is a stage when issues such as increasing visits to hospital and increasing medication will naturally occur. Changes in relationships, and the ability to work and cope independently also occur as does consideration of more practical issues such as care at home, care of any children – these are all issues as people become more unwell. Many patients obviously find this transition a difficult time and it is not unusual to experience symptoms of depression during this stage. However, for some patients it brings an end to uncertainty and many cope without further help and support (see Chapters 9 and 10).

During the terminal stages of HIV infection counselling again can be helpful, as this may be a time when the diagnosis is disclosed to more people. Discussion regarding death and dying, making of wills, and guardianship of children can be distressing at the time but may relieve anxiety once completed. Again counselling may be helpful to aid adaptation to increasing ill-health (see Chapters 9, 10 and 11).

After someone has died, bereavement counselling may be helpful for those who are left behind, although this is not always necessary, particularly if people have supportive family and friends. One feature of HIV infection is that for some groups multiple bereavement is commonplace, for example among homosexual men, injecting drug users and people from countries where HIV is very common such as parts of Africa. In such groups, some of those who 'survive', whether or not they too have HIV, may experience 'survivor's guilt'.

Staff burnout

While much of this book is about the patient or the person with HIV infection, it is plain that health care professionals need to be alert to the complexities of HIV infection without needing to understand the exact details. Looking after people with HIV and getting to know their partners and families can be very stressful.

One issue which is becoming more prominent, perhaps as a result of increasing workload, ever-increasing expectations and the inevitable resource constraints, is staff burnout. Perhaps as a result of looking after a group of young people with a life-threatening condition, or one that is as yet without cure, caring for people with HIV and AIDS can be stressful. As has been mentioned previously, stigma because of sexuality, drug-use, different and diverse lifestyles has meant that often the person does not always have a traditional family support system. This inevitably means that health care professionals perhaps begin to form part of the informal care network, especially if the person develops advanced disease. Another factor worth mentioning is that patients with HIV and AIDS can suffer with mental illness either directly from HIV infection or secondary to subtle changes within the brain. The exact prevalence of this latter process is unknown though the most serious manifestation, that is dementia, is thankfully rare (see Chapter 3).

What, therefore, is burnout? Burnout is a syndrome characterised by 'demoralisation and decompensation' along with feelings of irritability, anxiety and depression (King 1993). Other features may be the onset of physical symptoms (headaches, nausea, aches and pains, decreased appetite) and also a feeling of indispensability, rudeness to colleagues, neglect of social life and of course a worrying dependence on alcohol, cigarettes and other more noxious drugs. Insight can be lost in the process. The cause of all these is the sustained pressure – usually at work – leading to the feelings described above. It is a syndrome that is common to people who are in 'people-skills' jobs, for example those in the health professions, local authorities and other vocations.

One of the best ways of avoiding burnout is firstly to acknowledge that it exists. Although this sounds fairly glib it is fundamental to the process of developing insight into what can be a painful process. Certainly for doctors, arguably it is this lack of insight which has partially resulted in the profession continuing to suffer with higher rates of suicide, alcoholism, drug abuse, poor marriages and dysfunctional relationships than the average population. It is almost impossible to tease out exactly why these occur more frequently in doctors than in the average population. Nevertheless, there is something about the health-related professions that attracts high-achievers, is undoubtedly pressured and involves a certain emotional process that comes from looking after people in a clinical arena. Perhaps the answer to how to prevent burnout is relatively simple: take regular breaks, including holidays and study-leave, leave work on time, expect to fail sometimes, ask for help from senior colleagues or your general practitioner, and realise once and for all that no one is indispensable.

Boundaries

Clearly many health professionals find caring for people with HIV infection and AIDS stressful. One particular feature in HIV and AIDS care is that often both health care professional and patient may share certain characteristics, for example age group, sexuality and lifestyle. Interestingly, this may be similar to the vocation of general practice where patients often talk about their doctor as if 'they are a friend more than a doctor'.

Where this may become problematic is when the clinician–patient boundary is blurred. This may have implications for many aspects of the relationship such as prescribing, further follow-up, and future plans, especially if the patient deteriorates. Perhaps an early phase of this process may be an over-dependence on the part of the patient towards the doctor or nurse. This is a complex problem since it brings to the fore the question of who is more dependent on whom: is the patient more dependent on the health care professional (the orthodox view) or is it vice-versa (the need to care)? Of course this creates an instant practical problem because if the health professional is away on holiday or study-leave the patient is suddenly bereft of the emotional support. In order to prevent this it is wise to introduce the patient to other members of the team for such instances. *It should never be the case that any member of the team is irreplaceable.*

One of the more stressful clinical aspects for doctors and nurses is looking after people who continually return to them seeking help, advice or reassurance (King 1993). This subject cannot be fully explored here but it clearly has significant implications for health care workers. Patients who return to the doctor continually for whatever reason over a period of weeks, months or years are sometimes called 'frequent-attenders'. In general practice these frequent-attenders are often noted for their 'thick files' and it is common for such a group to have been referred to many agencies, both in the community but more likely to hospital specialists. This group of patients is very mixed and equally challenging to health care workers. This type of behaviour, of continually seeking help from doctors and nurses is sometimes associated with minor forms of mental illness – but not always.

References

Harrison, M.J.G. and McArthur, J.C. (1995) *AIDS and Neurology*, Edinburgh: Churchill-Livingstone.

King, M. (1993) *AIDS, HIV and Mental Health*, Cambridge: Cambridge University Press.

Miller, R. and Madge, S. (1996) Chapter 16 'The place of counselling in the prevention, diagnosis and management of HIV infection' in *AIDS. A Pocket Book of Diagnosis and Management*, Mindel, A. and Miller, R. (eds), second edition, London: Arnold Publishing, Oxford University Press.

6 The General Practitioner and the Primary Health Care Team

Having provided information on various disciplines and how they can help people with HIV infection and AIDS, it is only appropriate that the clinical team in the community is described. Many of these, for example the physiotherapist or the occupational therapist, have already been mentioned in Chapter 4. The majority of the services they provide are accessible through a general practitioner (GP).

The structure of general practitioner (GP) services can be variable – as a result, this chapter is presented as a series of questions which people most commonly ask of their primary care services. Although many of these questions are not specifically about HIV and AIDS, many of the issues will be discussed with HIV/AIDS in mind, for example see the question on confidentiality on p. 99.

Can I register with any GP?

Unfortunately not. The way the system works is that general practitioner services – this will be expanded upon shortly – are organised around a particular locality or area. Unfortunately again, these localities are rarely fixed and defined, thus they do not usually correspond to known boundaries (for example borough or town). This does mean, however that by and large most practices will be flexible. The way to find out is to enquire at a local practice or health centre.

What is the difference between a health centre and a practice?

This is confusing to many people, many of whom are health workers! A general practice may consist of many partners and can be housed in a variety of settings of which a health centre is an example. Thus, health centres are merely buildings which contain many services, such as doctors, nurses, dentists, counsellors, chiropodists and sometimes, complementary therapists.

Usually a big difference between a health centre and a specially constructed GP surgery is that the health centre rooms are rented by the doctors who are housed therein. A specially built and designed GP surgery may well be entirely owned by the GPs. Other terms for a GP practice may include GP surgery, GP consulting rooms, health centre or a GP office (rare and more North American).

Latterly, more and more general practitioners are working as partners. The most common size of partnership is four to five partners. The single-handed doctor is seen by many in the medical profession as old-fashioned. However, as far as patients are concerned, the tendency is for the smaller partnerships to be more friendly and caring. In many ways, especially in larger towns, it is the patient's choice to choose a larger practice or a small, friendlier practice.

It should therefore be clear that many health centres contain within them one or more general practitioner partnerships. For example, a medium-sized centre may contain a single-handed doctor and two other small partnerships. Confusingly, these partnerships are entirely separate and autonomous. In other words, the only commonality is that they all share the premises of the one health centre. As far as registering with a particular practice is concerned, each must be regarded as independent of each other.

What if I do not like my current GP?

Change your general practitioner. It is important to state here that, of course, you may not like the next GP either! One fair strategy is to give your doctor 'two strikes', thus if the first encounter was not to your liking, make another appointment and try again (doctors are only human too!).

In 1990, the process whereby patients could change from one doctor to another was significantly simplified. Hence all patients need do is approach another GP practice and if the practice is willing to 'register' the patient, the patient simply signs the appropriate form (called the FP1). These arrangements mean that patients do *not* have to seek permission to leave their old practice.

When patients register with a new doctor, they will be simply asked who their previous doctor was in order that the notes can be obtained from the respective health authority. This means that theoretically the same set of notes follows the patient throughout their life, something which is usually advantageous.

Although choice has been mentioned above, it is clear that if you live in a small village or town, your choice may not be so large. Quite simply the surgery in your town may be the only one for miles, in which case choice does not exist.

In larger towns or cities it may be that all the practices in a particular health centre have a working policy that patients are not allowed to transfer from one practice to another. While this appears to be rather inflexible, the theory behind it is that a number of patients may have continually transferred from one practice to another within the health centre. This is usually bad for patients since there is no 'continuity of care' and it tends to be an administrative nightmare for all practices.

The way around this problem, especially if you would definitely like to register with a particular practice is to see that practice's manager and explain why you would like to join. This sounds rather like 'having to interview' the practice, however it may be useful in the situation where there is an official bar to transferring from one practice to another within the same health centre.

Although it may be difficult to change practices in such circumstances, it is usually possible to see another doctor in the same practice even though you are officially registered with one particular doctor. The only exception to this guideline is where the practice operates a personal list, in other words it is only possible to see the doctor with whom you are registered on most or all occasions. This last arrangement is quite rare however.

What if I am new to an area and need to register with a GP, how do I go about finding a suitable one?

This is a difficult question since trying to find a suitable GP will depend on your particular requirements. For example do you want a GP who is a women, or who can speak French, or one that has an interest in a particular speciality, or (and this may be more difficult!) do you want all three? In reality many people opt for the nearest practice, almost irrespective of its size, its location and the doctor's interests.

If you are keen on finding the right GP a number of strategies are possible. Thus, getting to know the area is an obvious first step, although this may take some time and registering with a GP is important. One very useful source of information is the 'practice leaflet'. Many practices now produce a leaflet which outlines a number of points about the particular practice. For example, it should name the partners of the practice and surgery times. It may also describe the clinical interests of the individual partners. The practice leaflet will state how to access the practice nurse and also the nurse practitioner (see later this chapter) if available within the practice, and may describe how to access other services in the locality and provide simple health advice for common complaints.

Importantly the practice leaflet may include a written 'non-discrimination policy' which has been shown to highlight the more progressive partnerships in this field of HIV and AIDS (Shaw et al. 1996). Thus, the surgery may also state their position on confidentiality, which is especially important in this area of clinical practice, and their document should also outline the procedure on how to register a complaint, details of which have changed in the last few years. If in doubt about this the practice manager would be a useful member of the team to approach.

Another option when looking for the right practice is to seek the advice from a local chemist since they receive prescriptions from all the surrounding practices. Although it will be rare for the chemist to recommend a particular practice, they may well point out the range of practices in the area.

Finally, a more formal way of choosing a practice is to seek out written information from local libraries or contact the local health commission. Usually a list of practices will be available in the library and these often state the size of the practice, the names of all the partners, the times of surgeries, the availability of special clinics and the particular interests of the doctors. This type of list is very useful and well worth seeking out.

What does a 'closed list' mean?

Although this is not an official term, some practices will state their list is temporarily closed, in other words they are not registering new patients. Thus, you may be in the unfortunate position of having identified a practice that will not register you because their list is closed. The reasons for closing a list may be multiple and complex, however, a primary reason might be that a practice may feel they do not have the resources to care for an increasing number of patients. There is little that can be done about this;

however, if you feel this is unfair then you could try to make an appointment to see the practice manager.

If you really thought that 'the closure of the list' was being operated in a discriminatory fashion, then you would be advised to seek the help of the local Community Health Council (CHC), the name of which is usually obtainable from the local telephone directory or from the Citizen's Advice Bureau (CAB).

What other services are available alongside GP service?

The list of services is endless and clearly the exact details will depend on your particular GP location and premises to some extent. The most obvious of all the aligned services – usually other primary care services – are the nursing services including district nurse services, midwifery, health visitors and sometimes school nurse services. One exception to this may be the practice nurse, who is usually employed by the practice and her role is defined by health promotion and prevention tasks. These in turn are usually prioritised by the practice as a whole including the practice nurse. Thus the practice nurse may be responsible for the management of cervical smears and the 'flu-jab' campaign and in some surgeries is responsible for sexual health promotion clinics, contraception and other special diabetes or asthma clinics. The practice nurse tends to be more practice-based, thus home visits are few and infrequent, though again this is ultimately dependent on the type of practice.

Some practices will have physiotherapy and other therapy services (occupational therapy, speech therapy) either on-site or will have access to such services in the locality (see Chapter 4). Other services located in the health centre may also include chiropody and perhaps social service-type clinics where the focus in on welfare rights and housing advice.

What is a nurse practitioner?

In many progressive practices it is possible to see either a practice nurse, nurse practitioner or a doctor. How do you decide which is the most appropriate professional for you on a particular occasion? And what is the difference between a practice nurse and a nurse practitioner? Once again the answer here is dependent on your reason for seeking help. As stated above, the main tasks of the practice nurse are focused on particular health promotion and prevention schemes, for example cervical smears, or hypertension (high blood pressure) monitoring. The practice nurse often works from mutually agreed guidelines and if there are problems which fall outside such guidance then these are referred to the doctor.

A nurse practitioner is a relatively new type of nurse who is more of an independent nurse clinician. She or he is often very well qualified having completed midwifery and health visiting training and they represent another skilled member of an integrated primary care team. Nurse practitioners, like midwives for example, can prescribe certain medications, usually from a limited list or formulary. The types of areas where nurse practitioners may help in any one practice include seeing 'emergency patients', managing minor illnesses, providing a service complementary to the GPs and referring patients to specialist colleagues. Of course the training implications for this type of staff member are not insignificant to the practice, though the potential benefits to patients is the rightful spur to the development of such posts.

What is a clinical trials nurse?

Very occasionally a practice will have a specially designated clinical trials nurse, though this type of nurse, who is responsible for the co-ordination, surveillance and organisation of clinical trials, is more commonly based in hospital units. In the sphere of HIV and AIDS treatment, especially in the larger centres, this type of nurse, who is extensively trained, will have their own clinics and will also be liaising with clinic doctors. They have a particular role in ensuring that all concerned with the trial such as the doctor, laboratory personnel and pharmacists all work in unison. In addition they provide a critical link between the clinic and the pharmaceutical company.

Are all the GP's services free?

By and large yes, though there are important exceptions. This may sound rather pedantic but most health care costs are paid for through taxes, thus they are far from free. In addition certain primary care charges, for example optician and dental service, are normally paid for, though these tend to be dependent on earnings and the receipt of certain benefits. It is also wise to acknowledge that prescriptions are paid for – and these are for each item on the prescription. For those with some conditions such as diabetes (insulin-dependent only) or hypothyroidism, prescriptions are free and this then covers all items.

The provision of private letters and certificates are one aspect of GP services which needs to be mentioned since it causes endless amounts of confusion. A GP's work consists of what is termed 'general medical services' (GMS). Thus, where a private certificate is required or a private medical examination is undertaken, a fee is payable to the doctor because such duties fall outside the remit of general medical services. Most practices will have a list of charges made for such procedures. Again if you are unsure then ask at the reception for this list.

Lastly, though related to the above point, if you wish to see a private specialist then you can expect your GP to write a referral letter, as this would be the case for an ordinary National Health Service (NHS) specialist opinion. There should be *no* charge to the patient for writing this referral letter.

What can I expect once I have registered?

Again the variability of general practices will inevitably mean that one patient's experiences may not be the same as another even though both live in the same part of the country. Usually, however, practices offer new patients a one-off 'health check', which may well be carried out by the practice nurse. There is not too much to this except it allows the practice to identify need while ensuring that 'lifestyle' parameters such as smoking and drinking are recorded (and hopefully acted upon) in the notes.

There has been much adverse publicity about confidentiality in general practice being not as robust as in other places such as hospitals. This may have arisen from studies in the mid-1980s which identified the attitudes of a group of GPs as being rather negative and judgmental, especially towards people who were gay or using drugs. This evidence is now old and certainly 'alternative lifestyles' appear to be accepted with greater readiness than in previous times.

Confidentiality in practice is a very serious matter. The extent to which confidentiality is protected ought to be as good if not better than in the hospital sector. Your GP will regard everything you say as confidential, unless there is very good evidence – which would need to be presented if it was questioned – that someone was going to be harmed by maintaining this as confidential.

Of course, the question of providing third parties with information is very relevant here, such as insurance or life assurance companies. Forms provided by such companies often need to be filled out by the GP if and when the applicant applies for a mortgage or when a life insurance policy is taken out. It is prudent to note that these forms can only be filled out where the applicant has given consent. In fact the GP cannot divulge any information about any aspect of the patient's condition without explicit and informed consent. The difficulty here is that patients sometimes do not appreciate that their consent (that is, their signature) can mean that a substantial amount of information may be passed to the company without the full realisation of the applicant. The question therefore arises: what if I register with a GP and there is sensitive information about which I may not want to go into my notes?

Again this is difficult; however, you have a right to be concerned, especially in these days of computerised notes and 'paperless practices' (which in reality do not exist). One obvious way of confronting this problem is to ask what is being recorded in the notes. In the majority of cases, the GP will be pleased to explain this further and sometimes a mutually acceptable way of recording particularly sensitive information in the notes is the only way forward. Many doctors adopt the British Medical Association policy of referring questions back to the insurance company when they ask the GP about the 'patient's lifestyle'. In fact many practices have a ready-made stamp which states the following in all such mortgage and insurance policy forms: *'It is essential that a doctor does not speculate about the patient's lifestyle or "risk" of HIV infection. Such questions can only be answered by the patient and the life insurance company should be directed to seek the information from the patient him/herself'*.

It is important to acknowledge here that since the 1988 Access to Medical Records Act it is the right of all patients to see their notes. In general practice a request like this needs to be put in writing and practices can make a small charge for the issuing of the notes.

Patients cannot take the notes away, no matter how much or little information is contained therein. All clinical notes, including hospital or Trust notes belong to the Secretary of State for Health. Thus the relevant pages of sheets can be copied but the hard copy cannot be taken away.

Can I obtain free condoms from my GP?

As in previous answers there is no set answer here because all practices differ. In many metropolitan cities sexual health promotion is now a large-scale activity and hence practices may be participating in schemes which encourage condom distribution. How this is done is again variable. The last thing practices want is for condoms to be distributed without the attendant 'health promotion' which should accompany it, for example, do people know how to use them? (Don't forget there is now a female condom, see Chapter 2.) Moreover, condoms ought to be given out with the appropriate lubricant. Lubricated condoms, used with a spermicide, can be a very effective form of contraception. In cases where a pregnancy may be disastrous for the woman, a double form of protection may be appropriate, for example, the contraceptive pill and a condom (see Chapter 1). The point here is that a request for condoms is followed up by a frank discussion about other sexual health promotion issues.

One of the main reasons for the current attention about sexual health promotion is that other sexually transmitted diseases, such as chlamydia, are becoming more common. The need for widespread education and raised awareness about these more insidious, but less emotive infections is more important than ever before.

Another option for people wanting contraceptive and sexual health advice is to visit 'family planning clinics', admittedly a rather out-dated term for such clinics. These clinics which are often housed in the same health centres provide another set of outlets for obtaining free condoms and general advice. One advantage for such clinics is that opening times are suited to particular types of women. Thus women with child care needs can attend the mid-afternoon clinics, while women returning late from work may be able to attend special early evening clinics where these are available.

In larger cities, another service – called the Brook clinics – specialise in providing such advice (including what to do if a young person finds herself pregnant) for younger people (teenage–23 years).

What if I am too ill to go to the surgery?

This is another difficult question, although the answer ought to be clear. An explanation is first necessary.

General practitioners know that it is simply much more efficient to encourage patients to attend the doctor in surgery. This is so even where there are no further appointments available (doctors can usually find a way of fitting in emergency patients!). However, GPs also realise that sometimes a patient, usually an adult, may be too ill to attend, in which case a home visit is entirely necessary. In terms of organisation, and this clearly depends on the type of practice, 'home visits' are carried out towards the end of the morning. In larger practices where there is a designated doctor to do the home visits these may be done earlier in the day.

Sometimes patients perceive (wrongly) that their illness, for example, a sore throat and fever, does not allow them out of the house. This misperception is particularly common in the case of young children. While this is not totally unreasonable, it is always better to try and attend surgery because the chances are that you will be seen sooner. In addition the surgery has all the right instruments for further care (for example investigations) and the full range of primary care staff is at hand. Finally, it is far more cost-efficient for as many people as possible to be seen in surgery rather than at home.

What happens if an emergency occurs out-of-hours?

Up until recently it was common for many GPs, if not most, to 'cover' the patients from their own surgeries on a rota basis, perhaps once or twice per week. GPs have a contract with the government to provide general medical services 24 hours per day, seven days per week, and 52 weeks per year and as such the out-of-hours arrangements are critically important.

Recently, especially in cities (though spreading to rural areas), doctors from large localities have banded together to form co-operatives (co-ops for short). These work to provide comprehensive cover to many practices in the same locality using the local doctors.

However, because of an economy of scale, each individual doctor may need to work a few hours extra per month, which, in contrast to previous arrangements, is a major reduction in the overall time 'on-duty'. The disadvantage to patients is that they are likely to see a different GP from their usual doctor. However, even previously many GPs did not cover the nights they were supposed to, instead they employed 'deputies' who provided cover for the practice.

The other major change in this newer system is that, in the cities especially, this new out-of-hours service usually has consulting rooms which it uses to the maximum. Thus patients with an emergency will be persuaded, for reasons stated earlier, to attend the new centre where the patient can be investigated, treated and managed accordingly. Of course where this is not possible the patient will be visited at home. In the most efficiently run systems, details of any patients visited or treated at the emergency centre will be faxed through to the patient's own surgery by the following morning.

What does 'shared care' for patients with HIV/AIDS mean?

The problem with the concept of shared care is that no single definition exists which adequately satisfies the many dynamic stakeholders involved. In addition health professionals often talk about shared care as if there was only one meaning, despite there being many different models. This is not the right context for exploring this topic comprehensively, however, a few basic points will be highlighted (see Mansfield and Singh 1993).

'Shared care' was an attempt to re-balance care for people with HIV infection and AIDS in the late 1980s in the most affected areas, such as London and Edinburgh. There were many reasons for this including what was then an impending epidemic and a feeling that secondary care (hospitals and clinics) was becoming unnecessarily prominent in the overall care of people with the HIV infection (Pinching 1989). This last point should be seen in the context that, though the hospital clinics had responded first, could the ever-increasing demand for such prime services be sustained? Lastly, there was an unmistakable feeling that general practitioners were merely a limited resource in the overall care of people with HIV infection and AIDS. Therefore several small initiatives around the country were devised to try and reverse some of these trends (Mansfield and Singh 1993).

The question arose whether HIV infection and AIDS were any different to any other serious, life-threatening condition where in the majority of circumstances, patients only accessed specialist care through their general practitioner.

The specific question about shared care arose because there have been other successful examples of shared care (for example antenatal care) where pregnant women carry their own notes, models also followed in diabetes care and increasingly in asthma care. Such a process was aided by the greater propensity to sharing notes and certainly allowing a patient access to their notes.

In certain Scottish cities there has always been a greater involvement of primary care professionals in HIV and AIDS. Thus, shared care signifies care which is shared between the primary and secondary care sectors in line with many conditions such as those mentioned above. Another component of this is that clinical decisions are shared between all parties, including first and foremost the patient. What this certainly means is that communication – which is a vital aspect of this shared ethos in care (Guthrie and Barton 1995) – is regular, consistent and purposeful.

In a valiant attempt to try and explore this further, hospital units in West London conducted a formal study 'combining specialist and primary care teams' involving patients with HIV and AIDS (Smith et al. 1996). Their results were fascinating and a brief synopsis is presented below.

First, the hospital units, based in West London, committed themselves to the study and the task of liaising with 88 general practitioners (GPs) in 72 practices in the locality. As part of this process, an HIV/AIDS management and treatment manual was devised, there were quarterly meetings for all concerned and a regular newsletter was produced.

Second, 'fax units' were provided to those practices without one, and finally, all the study GPs could access the senior specialist for advice and help at all hours through a 24-hour mobile phone service number.

Once this infrastructure was in place, the main aim of the study was to 'develop and evaluate a model of health care for patients with HIV infection which integrated hospital based care with the services that are already provided and delivered effectively by primary health care teams' (Smith et al. 1996). The study looked at data both retrospectively (for the previous year) and prospectively (for two-and-a-half years).

The results were relatively dramatic for such a small study. The average length of a hospital in-patient stay was halved for those patients who had participated in the project for two years or more. Additionally the average number of visits to the out-patient clinic per month fell for patients with AIDS. On the other hand there was a substantial increase in the number of visits to GPs by patients with symptomatic HIV and AIDS.

A small section of GPs were sent questionnaires about the study and they felt that their working knowledge of HIV/AIDS had improved as had their confidence in managing patients with fairly complex problems. They attributed this enhanced proficiency to the regular communication which had occurred through the study. Importantly, they also felt that they could refer to hospital more appropriately, in other words refer on those patients whom they could not deal with themselves. At the same time a small number of patients were asked to give their views on the study and 60 per cent of respondents agreed that their care had improved.

Box 6.1   Key messages from the study 'Combining specialist and primary health care teams' (Smith et al. 1996)

- Too much health care for patients with HIV infection is provided by hospital-based teams.
- GPs make an important contribution to the care of this group of patients.
- While hospital clinics visits fell, those to GPs increased substantially.
- The average length of a hospital inpatient stay was reduced by 50 per cent.
- Simple, prompt and regular communication systems are necessary for a successful partnership between hospital and primary care teams.

Case history: KT

KT is a 27-year Spanish woman who has advanced HIV infection as reflected in her cytomegalovirus (CMV) retinitis and relatively recent pneumocystis carinii pneumonia (PCP). She is taking a cocktail of medications which she is managing extremely well and she attends the hospital clinic every month.

She was first diagnosed with HIV infection some eight years ago when she presented to the clinic with persistent generalised lymphadenopathy (including large lymph glands in her neck). At the time she was suspicious she was HIV-positive because of a history of injecting drugs during her teenage years though on an intermittent basis only. She admitted to 'sharing works' during this time. At the time of diagnosis, her partner, Chris, was also tested and found to be negative. Despite this, KT and Chris are now married and they live near the hospital unit in London. KT has given up all street drugs. Both Chris and his family are extremely supportive of KT. Her family visit regularly from Spain.

KT is fully aware of her poor prognosis and has already made a will and has gone so far as to arrange her funeral.

She is linked in with community services including a nurse specialist and her general practitioner, both of whom visit in her home. KT and her husband live in an adapted house on the ground floor of a block of flats. She has made a good initial response to a change in her anti-viral combination therapy although she still experiences some adverse effects from the medications including nausea, sickness and headaches. Her aim is to be well enough to attend her sister's wedding in Spain in about six months' time.

KT presents few problems. She is relatively 'compliant' with the medication and also her hospital appointments. She is personable and well-organised and has support from her husband, a close group of friends and family. Thus her use of hospital and community support services is not as great as it could be. She is unusually aware of her vulnerable circumstances and, if worried, presents to doctors early in the course of any episode. Psychologically she is well-adjusted to her diagnosis and has made the relevant plans should her overall health deteriorate. She also has realistic short-term goals: she has set her heart on seeing her younger sister married next year in Spain and she admits this is 'keeping her going'. She is thus very keen to remain well, in other words she is taking her medication as instructed and trying her best to follow the advice of the primary care team and the specialist clinic.

For their part, the hospital specialists are well-aware that KT supports herself the majority of the time and treat her accordingly. They are keen to let the GP play his full part in her care and thus they fax any significant changes to the medication regime after each visit to the clinic. They also alert the GP to special precautions with other medications (antibiotics for example) especially in view of her new and complex regime.

References

Guthrie, B. and Barton, S. (1995) 'HIV at the hospital/general practice interface: bridging the communication divide', *International Journal of STD and AIDS*, 6: 84–88.

Mansfield, S. and Singh, S. (1993) 'Who should fill the care gap in HIV disease?' *Lancet*, 342: 726–8

Pinching, A.J. (1989) 'Models of clinical care'. *AIDS*, 3 (suppl. 1): S209–S213.

Shaw, M., Tomlinson, D. and Higginson, I. (1996) 'Survey of HIV patient's views on confidentiality and non-discrimination policies in general practice', *British Medical Journal*, 312: 1463–4.

Smith, S., Robinson, J. Hollyer et al. (1996) 'Combining specialist and primary health care teams for HIV positive patients: retrospective and prospective studies', *British Medical Journal*, 312: 416–20.

7 The Hospital Team

Hospitals can seem daunting and somewhat confusing institutions to anyone. Levels of anxiety in those attending as patients are often understandably raised.

In this section the aim is to explain the roles and responsibilities of several health professionals the patient may encounter in the hospital, either as an in-patient or an out-patient. Often, as in the last chapter, the roles of some of these professionals are not specific to HIV. Each hospital will have a slightly different 'set-up' and a range of professionals that can be accessed for treatment and advice. However, broadly speaking what follows is a description of the most commonly accessed health care workers within a context of HIV and AIDS, their specific roles and what can be expected from them.

Doctors

Setting

Some HIV treatment centres are based in Genito-Urinary Medicine (GUM) or Sexually Transmitted Disease (STD) clinics and others are based in other sub-specialities such as Chest Medicine, Infectious Diseases and Haematology. This is because HIV is a relatively new disease and it did not always fit into existing specialities. In addition in some hospitals genito-urinary clinics were not established.

Out-patient clinics usually take place in a well-defined unit within a hospital. Investigations, including different 'tests', take place in a variety of departments usually dotted around a hospital. A patient may find they need to get to know their way around a hospital in some detail.

If a person needs to be admitted to hospital for several days (in-patient) they may stay on a designated ward where the staff are very familiar with HIV-related problems. In some such wards not every patient will have HIV in order to avoid that ward becoming known as 'the HIV ward', because some people do not want their visitors to know about their HIV status. It is also likely that non-HIV patients will be on the same ward because of the general shortage of beds and the number of 'emergency' patients being admitted at any one time.

If an individual with HIV infection is admitted to hospital as an emergency, they may initially be placed on a ward where the staff are less expert in HIV medicine. These wards will invariably have contact with the staff from the more recognised HIV wards in order to ensure quality of overall care.

Hierarchy

One of the more baffling things that patients, friends and families have to cope with within the hospital setting is the hierarchy of doctors. The following is a description of a standard hierarchy in the UK.

A *consultant* is the head of a team of doctors and usually other health care workers. In some hospitals there will be several consultants who look after patients with HIV infection and in other hospitals the service may be managed by one consultant. Consultants are doctors who have had many years of training and are experienced in their specialist field of medicine.

They see patients in clinics, but as they are the head of the team they are often in most demand. Most consultants try to see patients at some of their hospital visits, but it may be impossible to see them every time. Nowadays consultants increasingly have other work commitments that can encroach into the time they have to see patients.

A *senior lecturer* is an experienced doctor who also has an additional teaching role. They are a university as well as a hospital appointment. In practical terms a senior lecturer and a consultant are the same entity, the former however has additional teaching commitments.

Senior registrars are the next most senior doctors in the medical team. They often work in a hospital for several years before they move on to a consultant post, and may be involved in research as part of their training. This activity is expected of senior registrars prior to their becoming consultants.

Registrars are the next step in the hierarchy. These doctors are often the middle-grade doctors who spend time liaising between the junior doctors (who are on the wards), the consultant and the patients. They are often present on hospital wards and they will generally have daily contact with such patients. They will also attend clinics in the out-patient's department.

Registrars tend to train in any one hospital for six months to two years, thus they move fairly frequently between specialities and different hospitals. Registrars will usually have attained further post-graduate qualifications in whatever they choose as their speciality.

Senior house officers are doctors who have been qualified for one to four years. They are often part of a team for six months to a maximum of two years and often deal with patients both on the wards and in the clinics. Senior house officers will probably be deciding which speciality they would like to pursue, or may have done this and be working towards the post-graduate qualifications mentioned in the last section.

House officers are doctors who have completed five years' undergraduate training. They generally work on wards and have much less to do in out-patient clinics. As house officers, doctors have to undertake one year in either general surgery or general medicine and as part of their medical training they may cover HIV as a speciality.

There are other doctors who are often an integral part of the team who do not quite fit into this hierarchy such as *staff grade physicians*, *associate specialists* and *clinical assistants*. These are doctors who may not work full time or work in different specialities. They are often experienced but for one reason or another (in the past domestic arrangements were a major barrier to successfully pursuing any medical career), work in the team over an extended period of time.

Continuity

The previous paragraph alludes to one of the main problems in medicine for a patient, that is one of continuity of care. Doctors move around frequently in their jobs and their training, although this may change in the future. Patients may not see the same doctor for a sustained period. Once again this is not peculiar to HIV, and is one of many good reasons for having a general practitioner (GP) who may be able to provide that continuity. Other patients would like their GP to be more expert in aspects of HIV and AIDS although this is not always possible. Some patients find GPs a useful 'sounding board' to discuss HIV-related problems (see Chapter 6).

Consultants are the doctors that move the least but are the most difficult to see on a regular basis. When patients are seen either in casualty or on wards out-of-hours (including at weekends) they may be seen by a doctor who is less familiar with HIV-related problems. However, doctors now have specific training in HIV and would be familiar with management, treatment issues and emergency care procedures and thus this should not be a problem. It is important to remember that even at weekends, there is a consultant 'on-call' who may need to come into the hospital if there are difficult problems.

Doctors of all grades will have time out of work for holidays, study leave for exams or other training. Their work may be covered by 'locum' or 'stand-in' doctors.

Hospital referrals

Sometimes, for a variety of reasons, HIV doctors may request an opinion from a consultant in another sub-speciality in the hospital. These doctors may be very experienced in respect to HIV-related matters and are an integral part of service that any hospital offers. Listed below are some specialists to whom people with HIV are commonly referred.

Strategies for maximising the effectiveness of the consultation

People with HIV will visit doctors at varying frequencies when they are well. It may be only necessary to visit once every six months; however, when patients are more ill they may visit as regularly as every week. More specifically, if someone is considering starting treatments, or needing to switch treatments, they may need to visit every two weeks or so for the first couple of months. This is to monitor for side-effects and make sure that the medication is working.

Clinics are often busy places and coming to clinics is a stressful enough event for most patients. Therefore, patients will often forget to ask doctors questions, which is frustrating for patients (and for doctors since clearly questions remain unanswered which may influence other aspects of care). Patients may therefore come away from their consultation feeling dissatisfied. Listed below are a few handy hints that may help make a consultation with a doctor more effective. This should improve satisfaction for both patient and for the doctor. It is consciously written from the patient's perspective and may go some way to try and improve the overall communication between both parties:

1   *If you have a worry then mention it.* Doctors cannot guess and they may make assumptions about what patients are worried about and what they are not worried about.
2   Make a *short list* of your priorities with either questions or points that you need to mention. Try not to make this too long: five points is a reasonable list (though this depends upon how complex they are), but

Table 7.1   The hospital team: the role of specialists

Specialist	Areas of specialist advice and treatment
Dermatologist	Specialist in skin
Gastreoenterologist	Specialist in the gastrointestinal system
Obstetrician and Gynaecologist	Specialist in women who are pregnant and women who have gynaecological problems
Paediatrician	Specialist in care of children
Oncologist	Specialist in people with cancers (of all types)
Opthalmologist	Specialist in care of the eyes
Neurologist	Specialist in the nervous system and brain disorders
Psychiatrist	Specialist in mental health-related problems
Oral Surgeon	Specialists who have trained both as dentists and doctors (surgeons) for facial and oral-related problems
Ear Nose and Throat Surgeon	Specialist in problems of the ears, nose and throat
Orthopaedic Surgeon	Specialist – always a surgeon – in bones and limb disorders
Haematologist	Specialist in problems of the blood

fifteen points is far too many that can be realistically covered in a consultation.

3 Plan to mention your main problem, be it a specific symptom or any major worry, *early on* in the consultation and not as you are leaving the room. This way it will receive the time it warrants.

4 *Bring someone else in with you if you can.* This is helpful because it means that someone can hear what the doctor says to you and they can remind you of things that you may have forgotten if you are on your own.

5 *Do not be embarrassed* to ask doctors any questions or to talk to them about difficult subjects such as sex, relationship difficulties or drug use. Most doctors in HIV are experienced and little shocks or surprises them. Their role is not to be judgmental but to help you. It is also important to remember that the doctor does not work alone but in a team and it may be that other issues such as relationship problems or illicit drug use may

be more appropriately managed by other members of the team such as a counsellor.

6   *If you have concerns about medication such as side-effects,* tell your doctor and if you are not taking any medication they have prescribed for you. Doctors are not able to guess whether you are taking medication. They may wrongly assume that you are taking pills that you are not. Similarly, if you are taking non-prescribed medication it is much better that the doctor knows in case of potentially harmful drug interactions.

7   The *time* doctors have available to them varies for each consultation. If someone is acutely unwell with physical symptoms then this inevitably becomes the focus of the consultation. However, people with HIV disease are often physically well and more time is spent in the consultation discussing new monitoring tests, advances in HIV treatments, relationship worries, stresses at work and many other issues. An effective and productive consultation for both doctor and patient does not mean that it has to be time-consuming. The consultation skills of the doctor, prior knowledge and relationship with the patient, and the presenting problems of a patient, means that every consultation is different.

8   If, as a patient, you are *unhappy* about a particular doctor it is better to deal with him or her directly; an alternative is to try and approach the consultant who is 'in charge' of your care. Either of these is better than merely hoping things may change or feeling that 'you don't want to make a fuss'. It is much better for you to try and consult with someone who you can relate to, and trust. Most hospitals have well-established complaints procedures if you feel you need to make a complaint.

9   Wherever possible try to see the same one or two doctors, although do not forget that doctors may leave or go on holiday, so it is best to get to know a few clinic doctors so that you are not over-reliant on one person.

10   Ask your clinic doctor to write to your general practitioner so that, even if you rarely see your GP, when you do he or she is up to date with how you are, whether you have had recent investigations or what treatments you are taking.

On occasions, doctors may have medical students sitting in with them – these are trainee doctors. You may feel you would prefer the student not to be there, in which case you should tell the doctor. It is very useful for students to learn from patients and if you feel able it is very helpful for their training to be present during consultations.

Nurses

Nurses have a key role in both out-patient and in-patient care. They play an important role in patient advocacy, helping patients with basic physical care and various clinical tasks such as blood-taking and administering drugs. Nurses will help co-ordinate patients' discharge from hospital and liaise with other disciplines to access resources. Nurses are present on wards at all times and thus play an important role in the psychological well-being of the patient; they are the most accessible professionals for visitors if they also need support. Many nurses are experienced in the field of HIV, especially those that work on the HIV/AIDS wards, and are a useful resource when discussing treatments.

Hierarchy

A similar hierarchy exists in the nursing profession as in the medical profession. *Student nurses* are trainee nurses who are often present on the ward setting to gain experience. Once a student nurse qualifies, she (and increasingly he) becomes a *staff nurse*. When a staff nurse has several years' experience they may be promoted to a *senior staff nurse* position. A *sister* (*charge nurse* if *male*) is a more senior post and will often be in charge of a ward.

Models of care

There are various models of care within the nursing profession based on the philosophy of the hospital. Many hospitals will run what is called the *named nurse system* when patients are in-patients. This means one named nurse, who should be easily identifiable to the patient, is responsible to a particular patient or patients, thus it is the responsibility of that nurse to ensure that care for a shift (which may be up to twelve hours) has been provided.

The named nurse may be the team leader and will therefore be in charge of several colleagues at any one time. This system should improve continuity of care for the patient during their stay in hospital.

Community liaison nurses (community nurse specialists)

These are usually senior (sister grade) nurses who work at the hospital/community interface. There are many community nurse specialists in HIV work, especially in areas where HIV is common, and they are an important link between the hospital and the community. Community liaison nurses too, are often able to perform various tasks such as taking blood and administering drugs and also have a key role in the teaching and training of others, especially district nurses. They tend to be most involved with patients when they become more unwell. Not all areas have Community Nurse Specialists and in some areas the District Nurses have been trained to cover this role (see Chapter 4).

Research nurses

There are research nurses who are often a sister or senior grade. Their role is to co-ordinate clinical trials often with research doctors. They often have a wide knowledge about drugs and side-effects and are a useful resource for patients for further information. Research nurses often attend international conferences, and may be the most up-to-date and accessible person to talk to regarding new treatments (see Chapter 6).

Physiotherapists

In some hospitals there will be specialist physiotherapists who specifically manage patients with HIV infection and AIDS. In other hospitals a general physiotherapist will cover the HIV service. Physiotherapists have had several years' training and are particularly helpful for patients with neurological problems in helping them improve their mobilisation with exercises or aids such as walking frames. They can also help with ordering wheelchairs. Physiotherapists can give carers useful advice on lifting and aiding mobilisation of people who are very unwell. Some patients who have chest-related diseases see the physiotherapist for advice and sometimes treatment. They are also able to give advice on exercise and may see patients who are currently well for general advice and guidance (see Chapter 4 for information on community-oriented physiotherapists).

Dieticians

As in the previous example, in some hospitals there will be a named HIV dietician; however, in other services a general dietician may also cover patients with HIV infection and AIDS. Dieticians are a useful resource to advise patients on healthy eating when they are well. They are also able to advise patients when they are becoming unwell and suffering symptoms such as weight loss, vomiting and diarrhoea. They can advise and often provide supplementary drinks to aid weight-gain. It is also often useful to discuss any diet that is perhaps more unorthodox with a dietician before embarking on a stringent dietary programme. It may be helpful to see a dietician if medication requires dietary restrictions, or needs special timing around meals (see Chapter 8).

When patients are more unwell dieticians may help supplement normal feeding with *naso-gastric tube feeding*, when a tube is passed through the nose via the gullet and into the stomach. A liquid feed which is high in calories is then passed through the tube into the stomach. This system is particularly helpful when patients have become more unwell and perhaps have suddenly experienced weight loss.

Patients who are even more seriously ill may need help with short- and long-term feeding. In some hospitals patients may need a small operation by which a tube is passed directly to the stomach from the skin outside. This is called a percutaneous endoscopic gastrotomy tube or a *PEG tube*. High-calorie feeds can be given this way, usually overnight. These have been effective in patients with advanced disease; however, this needs careful consideration prior to the decision since it is a fairly invasive procedure. Dieticians will usually liaise with community dieticians when people with complex dietary needs are based at home (see Chapter 4).

Occupational therapists

Occupational therapists may be based in the hospital or in the community. They can visit people at home and advise on adaptations in the home such as hand-rails, and specially equipped showers that make the home environment safer and more manageable for sick people (see Chapter 4 for further details).

Counsellors, psychologists and health advisers

Hospitals have different set-ups for patients to access counselling advice. Most will provide a service but many people choose more local services that are community based. Counsellors can help at all stages of HIV.

After HIV has been diagnosed, people may need support initially. Counsellors also may play a vital role in support as someone becomes more unwell. Generally speaking they prefer to take a pro-active role, in other words attempting to anticipate problems rather than waiting for crises to arise. However, sometimes it is impossible to predict a crisis or some patients prefer to wait until a crisis occurs to deal with the problem.

Counsellors will help people with HIV in their *decision making*, such as whether to continue at work, or telling friends, family and other relatives about their diagnosis. They can also provide advice on accessing benefits and housing needs, often through specific social services departments.

Counsellors and the above may act as sources of *referral* to other professionals when more specialist counselling or psychiatric support is deemed necessary. There are often many community-based counselling resources that counsellors in the hospital can advise for people with HIV to access. Some counselling services are helpful for partners, family and friends. However, it is very important to remember that most people have natural support networks from their partners, friends and family. Not everybody needs counselling and some people who would benefit from it do not want it! It is also questionable whether 'counselling' is objectively beneficial, though this is a topic which is highly controversial and dependent on several factors, none of which can be comprehensively examined in this text.

Welfare rights

People with HIV infection may be entitled to additional state benefits. Some hospitals will have members from the Citizen's Advice Bureau (CAB) available to discuss the pros and cons of seeking such benefits. Alternatively, people can see CAB members in the community and other organisations such as the Terence Higgins Trust also offer advice on benefits. For many patients it is clear, in the light of increasing ill health, that they are unable to work and sadly, seeking benefits is their only option.

However, it is important to not pressurise those who may be working into giving up work too early, as they may wish to continue working despite the fact that they are unwell. Some people have extremely sympathetic employers who will be flexible with work programmes. With the improved prognosis now for people with HIV infection, it is important to discuss all options, in the light of someone's symptoms, immunological results and current work situation, before making any decisions. In itself, seeking benefits may be a stressful and lengthy process.

People with HIV infection may need other advice such as help with re-housing applications; they may also need specific legal advice, perhaps because of disputes arising from issues related to their HIV status.

In addition, there is a group of patients, who are undoubtedly needy but who find it increasingly difficult to access care of any sort, that is, people seeking asylum in the UK. Many people with HIV infection in the UK are from abroad in areas where there is extreme political unrest (see case histories on pp. 139 and 143). Their most pressing problem may be that of seeking security to be able to stay in this country. This process is a lengthy and complex one where good relevant advice from especially trained solicitors is essential. There are such services available at agencies such as the Terence Higgins Trust and Immunity (see Appendix for further information).

The complexity and variety of benefits that one may be eligible for will not be covered in this book, as the benefit system is highly bureaucratic and infinitely complex, and one that is in a constant state of flux. The most appropriate advice in these circumstances is to try and access up-to-date information from a variety of reputable and professional sources including the ones mentioned in this sub-section.

Other team members

There are other critical disciplines within the HIV team with whom patients may not come directly into contact, for example *pharmacists*, who provide doctors with information on new drugs and have an in-depth knowledge on how best to take drugs, side-effects and drug interactions. Thus, doctors often view pharmacists as a major resource, especially in times of need! Pharmacists will dispense medication and give advice accordingly. In some hospitals they run special clinics advising on all aspects of medication (called 'compliance-clinics').

As with any other hospital team there is often a large behind-the-scene *administrative team* that is an integral and important resource. Wards and clinics also have *health care assistants* or *nursing auxiliaries* who are not clinically qualified but are often experienced members of the HIV team. People who have specific spiritual needs can meet with *religious representatives* in the hospital, and most hospitals have a chapel for patients or visitors to attend. *Hospital volunteers* can also be very helpful. Some wards and clinics also have access to *complementary therapists* who administer such therapies as massage, acupuncture and reflexology.

Hospital notes

All of a person's hospital records are kept in a set of notes. Some hospitals also have some information on computer. This information is confidential, but if you are concerned about who may have access to it and why, check with the hospital staff.

Changing hospital services

People may want to change their hospital services for a variety of reasons.

Sometimes people do not use their most local services initially. As they become more unwell, travelling long distances becomes problematic and they may choose to use more local services. People may also move house and thus may need to change services.

Doctors and nurses will have a good knowledge of other HIV services and can write to colleagues with information if a change in hospital is required. Historically in the UK, a small number of patients have chosen to 'shop around' to several different hospitals for their medical care. This may become more difficult in the future, and for reasons of continuity it is much better to remain with one hospital.

8 Drugs and HIV

The drugs that a person with HIV may be taking are extremely varied. The range of drugs is changing constantly with time, as new ones are being introduced which appear to be more effective. It can be very difficult for people to keep up-to-date with the newest, most effective drugs available. In the field of HIV and AIDS, new drugs are being developed almost more quickly than in any other field of medicine.

Different factors account for the variability of drugs that a person with HIV may take. *Patient choice* is the most important variable. Some people choose to take as many drugs as they are offered. Other people choose to take none at all. Most people find a balance that is right for them. There are complex reasons why people may choose to take or not to take drugs. The *side-effects* a person fears or has experienced may be worse than the perceived benefits of taking the drug. An individual's *personal* and *cultural beliefs* about how effective the drugs may be for them is an important influence. A good response to a drug will encourage someone to continue with it, either if they feel better or if their CD4 counts or viral load markers improve. The beliefs of the *doctors,* and their *relationship with the patient* and their *access* to certain drugs will also influence the drugs someone takes.

The *number of times a day* a drug has to be taken and any accompanying *special instructions* (for example should it be taken with certain foods?) will influence a patient. In addition, any drug interactions are also a factor here. For example Ganciclovir, a treatment against cytomegalovirus, must be taken three times a day on a full stomach; Indinavir must be taken three times a day on an empty stomach, which can mean pill-taking soon dominates someone's life. With some drugs, for example, the protease inhibitors' *compliance* is critically important. This means that drugs must be taken very stringently and no doses should be omitted. Taking medication

119

regularly, especially for some drugs such as the protease inhibitors, is very important since the virus can develop resistance to the drugs if they are taken erratically or irregularly. Some people are naturally more organised than others and can incorporate drug-taking into their daily routine.

External influences such as the *media* can influence drug-taking. Unfortunately the media often give out incorrect information. People panic and stop taking drugs if reports are bad, or they may feel angry if reports about a drug are promising but the drug cannot be easily accessed. The results of new *drug trials* and new drug combinations are reported rapidly and naturally can influence someone's decision as to when to start or change drugs. There are some very up-to-date and easily accessible sources of information on the newest drugs available (see the address at the end of this chapter). *Friends and family* can also influence drug taking and compliance.

The *progression* of HIV disease itself is important. Generally speaking, people who are well with good, intact, immune systems will be taking fewer drugs than those who have advanced AIDS-related problems. The number of drugs that people take tends to increase as they become more unwell and people with advanced disease may be taking a baffling number of complicated medications.

Drug formulation

Most drugs are given in tablet or liquid form. However, when people are particularly unwell and in hospital they may be given drugs through 'a drip', straight into a vein. Drugs are more effective when administered intravenously; however, by the same token, they often also have more side-effects. Sometimes people are discharged home taking drugs either in a drip or via a syringe driver (see p. 133). A more direct form of intravenous access is sought if someone needs intravenous drugs for a long time, in order to avoid their arms getting sore as many drips are used. This varies according to doctor and patient preference. Two of the commonest types are described below.

A *Hickman line* is a tube which connects to a large vein in the chest and an external tube with a connector and adapter which hangs on the chest wall. A *Port-A-Cath* is a small round rubber device which is buried beneath the skin and is attached to a large vein. A needle through the rubber connects to the vein. The advantage of this system is that it is less intrusive for the patient. With both of these systems, patients can learn to administer intravenous drugs themselves at home.

It is very important that doctors and other health care workers know exactly what drugs a person is taking. Some patients feel unable to disclose that they may be taking non-prescribed medications to their doctor. Similarly they may feel unable to tell the doctor that they do not want to be taking the drugs that the doctor is prescribing for them. It is much better for both doctor and patient that everyone knows exactly which drugs are being taken and when and why drugs may not be being taken. Once a drug has been prescribed for a patient it cannot be re-used for anyone else. The drugs used in HIV are often very costly, and if a patient is collecting drugs at home but not actually taking them, it is very wasteful. Doctors looking after patients with HIV fully understand why patients may not want to take medication and are very open to having discussions about medications. People may also take drugs that are not prescribed by doctors. These may be drugs that are commonly abused. Alternatively, drugs may be taken which are not prescribed by doctors but are either bought 'over-the-counter' (OTC) in pharmacies or are recommended by complementary practitioners. Doctors need to know exactly what is being taken and why. The cornerstone of any form of shared decision making around medications, especially in HIV and AIDS is *good communication between doctor and patient*.

Drugs taken in HIV disease can be broadly divided into four different groups:

1 They may be being taken to *prevent* specific infections.
2 There may be *anti-viral* drugs taken to reduce the HIV replication and preserve the immune system.
3 Drugs may be taken to counteract specific AIDS-related *infections*.
4 Drugs may be taken to counteract specific HIV and AIDS-related *symptoms*.

Drugs taken for prevention in HIV

Septrin (co-trimoxazole)

Septrin (co-trimoxazole) is a combination of two antibiotics which is given to people to prevent a type of pneumonia called pneumocystis carinii pneumonia (PCP). Doctors recommend patients take this when their immune system is becoming susceptible to PCP, usually when their CD4 counts are around 200 or if they are suffering several symptoms which are thought to be HIV related (see Chapter 3).

Septrin is an antibiotic which is effective in preventing PCP and also toxoplasmosis. It may also protect against other bacterial infections. One tablet of Septrin is taken every day, or three times a week if the patient is good at remembering to take a tablet on such a regime. It is very effective, cheap and generally well-tolerated in most patients. A small proportion of patients will be allergic to Septrin. This results in symptoms such as rash, headache and sickness often about ten days after starting Septrin. As Septrin is such an effective drug, doctors encourage patients who have a mild allergy to tolerate the transient symptoms or to try a desensitisation course of Septrin. Here they take Septrin in very low, but increasing doses, over a period of time (usually a week) to see if they can tolerate the drug. Often people who have had mild allergies to Septrin are therefore able to tolerate the drug after following the desensitisation course, which should only be undertaken under fairly close medical supervision.

Septrin does not influence the immune system and will not affect a person's T cell count. Because this antibiotic is a combination of two separate medications, there is no evidence that there is any resistance to Septrin. Hence, if an individual was unlucky enough to acquire PCP while taking Septrin (this is extremely rare if a patient is taking Septrin correctly) it could still be used as a treatment against the pneumonia, though in much higher doses usually.

Pentamidine

If someone is truly allergic to Septrin then the second line of treatment is pentamidine. It is given in a nebuliser form. This means inhaling particles of pentamidine through a compressed box similar to that which some asthmatics use. It needs to be given at least every month. Prior to inhaling the pentamidine most people are given a drug (terbutaline) which will open up the lung airways to make the pentamidine more effective. The whole process takes half an hour or so and can be done at home or in the hospital. Patients may cough when using the nebuliser, so if they are having the pentamidine in hospital it is advisable that a special, negative pressure room is used, in order to minimise any risk of other respiratory infections to other patients and members of staff. This is a particular concern with tuberculosis (TB), especially since multi-drug resistance TB is becoming more common (see Chapter 3).

One common side-effect of pentamidine is decreased blood sugar, so it is advisable to have had something to eat (a sandwich would suffice) prior to having the nebuliser.

There are also some other drug regimes that are occasionally used to prevent PCP.

Aciclovir

Aciclovir is a very safe and effective drug which is given to prevent recurrent attacks of herpes, something quite common in people with HIV disease.

Tuberculosis (TB)

TB is more common in someone who is also HIV-positive. People who are particularly susceptible to TB include those who have lived in areas where it is particularly prevalent, such as Africa or India. People who inject drugs or who may be homeless are also at particular risk from TB. Those who are particularly susceptible to TB are sometimes advised to take a drug to reduce the chances of contracting TB. The antibiotic isoniazid is often chosen since it is well-tolerated in most people.

Anti-viral drugs

Anti-viral drugs actually attack HIV and thus should boost the immune system. This should mean people will have less symptoms from HIV and will be less likely to develop any of the major opportunistic infections (Carpenter et al. 1996).

The history of anti-viral medication and HIV is somewhat chequered, mainly borne out of a frustration in both doctors and patients to find effective drugs very early when HIV was first identified. However, in the last few years great progress has been made. There are now several anti-viral drugs which are very effective in combating HIV infection and which have been shown in large studies to improve both the quantity and quality of people's lives. However, for a variety of reasons some patients still feel unsure about taking anti-viral drugs and are very reluctant to do so. This is changing as more and more effective drugs, with less side-effects, are now available.

AZT (Zidovudine) was the first drug that was used on its own in the mid to late 1980s to combat HIV infection. Latterly, results from large trials have shown that it is not very effective when used on its own in most patients. In the past, AZT was used in particularly high doses and people often experienced quite severe side-effects such as nausea and sickness, headaches and anaemia. Because of its lack of success and high profile of side-effects, many people were then reluctant to try subsequent anti-viral tablets and it is only in recent years that larger numbers of people are coming forward to use anti-viral drugs.

The available, commonly used anti-viral therapies are individually described below. This description provides basic information about the drug and practical advice about how it should be taken regularly and consistently. In addition their common side-effects and key drug interactions are described. All drugs have more than one name as they are often given an abbreviated name early on in their stages of development and then a more 'user-friendly' name later on. Where possible their abbreviated name is used.

Zidovudine (AZT, Retrovir)

AZT works by inhibiting the reverse transcriptase enzyme which the virus needs to replicate. AZT is available in capsules of 100mg, 250mg or a 300mg tablet. The usual dose is 250mg twice a day or 200mg three times a day. It is best taken either 8- or 12-hourly and should be taken with or after food. Its common side-effects include nausea and headaches, which often resolve after a few weeks. AZT may also cause muscle pains and, more seriously, suppression of the bone marrow which causes anaemia. When starting on AZT, or any other anti-viral medication, people are closely monitored so that side-effects can be observed and drugs either stopped, or switched if someone experiences severe side-effects. AZT and D4T (see later) should not be taken together because, in combination, their effects are antagonistic.

Didanosine (ddI/Didex)

ddI is also a nucleoside analogue like AZT and works similarly by inhibiting the HIV reverse transcriptase enzyme. It is normally taken at a dose of 200mg twice a day. However it is as effective if taken as a 400mg once a day dose. In people who weigh less than 60kg the dose is reduced to 125mg twice a day. Some people prefer to take ddI in one dose simply because it should be taken on a relatively empty stomach, that is either half an hour before food or two hours after food. Thus a once-daily dose for some is more convenient than a twice-daily dose.

The tablets need to be either chewed, which some people find unpleasant, or dissolved in water. They should not be mixed with Coca-Cola or orange juice. Common side-effects experienced with ddI include bloating and diarrhoea, nausea and vomiting and, very rarely, peripheral neuropathy, the latter is nerve damage to the extremities causing tingling, burning and sometimes numbness in the feet and occasionally the hands. Very rarely people may develop pancreatitis, a potentially very serious side-effect, which is an inflammation of the pancreas gland. This causes symptoms of severe abdominal pain and vomiting and anyone who experiences this shortly after starting on ddI should be seen in hospital where the relevant investigations can be initiated immediately.

Zalcitabine (ddC/Hivid)

This is also a nucleoside analogue that works by inhibiting the HIV reverse transcriptase enzyme. It is taken as a tablet three times a day at a dose of 0.75 microgrammes. There is no specific regime with respect to food. Common side-effects with ddC include nausea and vomiting, diarrhoea and peripheral neuropathy. It is however generally well-tolerated. Again, very rarely, it may cause pancreatitis.

Lamivudine (3TC/Epivir)

This too is a nucleoside analogue and works by inhibiting the HIV reverse transcriptase enzyme, therefore reducing HIV replication and allowing replenishment of CD4 cells. It is available as a tablet or a liquid at a dose of 150mg twice a day. There are no specific restrictions with respect to food and generally it is very well-tolerated with few side-effects. Some people experience headaches, nausea and vomiting, abdominal pains and diarrhoea and, very rarely, peripheral neuropathy. It does seem to have some action on the hepatitis B virus so is a good choice of drug in the small number of people who have persistent hepatitis B infection.

Stavudine (d4T/Zerit)

This is a nucleoside analogue and works by inhibiting the HIV reverse transcriptase enzyme. It comes as a capsule in a variety of strengths (15mg, 20mg, 30mg, 40mg). The normal dose is 40mg twice a day. However, in people who weigh less than 60kg, 30mg twice a day is used. In some people who already have peripheral neuropathy or hepatitis a lower dose (20mg twice a day) may be used to establish how well they tolerate the drug and monitor side-effects. It is antagonistic with AZT and should not be used in combination with this drug. Its main side-effects include nausea, diarrhoea and bloated abdomen and it can also cause a peripheral neuropathy and, more rarely, a hepatitis. Generally it is quite well-tolerated.

Nevirapine (Viramine)

This is a new class of drug called a non-nucleoside reverse transcriptase inhibitor. It is not licensed in the UK but this is expected in 1998. It is available in a dose of 200mg twice a day. Because a rash is a common side-effect, it is recommended that when people start on Nevirapine they start on a dose of 200mg once a day for two weeks before the twice-daily dosage. Generally it is very well-tolerated; however, some people develop a rash which in most cases will gradually disappear. A small number of people may need to stop taking the drug if the rash is severe. Other side-effects include nausea and headache. Nevirapine does have some significant drug interactions especially with some antihistamines and commonly prescribed antibiotics such as erythromycin and Augmentin. Anyone on Nevirapine should receive a complete list of all the drugs that it may interact with so that this can be shown to any doctors.

Retonavir

Retonavir is a protease inhibitor (Bartlett 1996). These are a new type of drug which work by inhibiting the production of the packages of HIV that are released from infected cells. All protease inhibitors are relatively new drugs that have only been licensed in the UK since 1996. They seem to be extremely effective against HIV and have produced dramatic improvements in many people. There is no doubt that these are the drugs that have in particular contributed to the dramatic improvements in many patients with advanced HIV disease. It is largely due to using these drugs in combination that the significant decrease in major AIDS-related problems has been seen. However, this type of medication should still be used with caution since aspects of their use are uncertain and they have their own problems.

It is common practice for anti-viral drugs now to be used in combination. Most commonly, people take three drugs. However, it is not clear which three drugs are the most effective and drug trials continue to try and answer this question. What is clear, however, is that taking medication regularly is extremely important. As discussed earlier, one consequence of erratic drug-taking is that resistance is more likely to develop. It seems that there is some cross-resistance between some of the anti-viral medications, especially the protease inhibitors. This means that once one protease inhibitor has become ineffective then it is possible that subsequent protease inhibitors will not be effective. It is also likely that some people may, unfortunately, inherit an HIV virus that is particularly resistant to certain anti-viral medication. In the future we may be able to do more specific tests to investigate which particular drugs are likely to be effective in specific patients. However, these are not widely available at present. Nobody knows exactly how long they will remain effective for, but what does seem clear is that people who are on protease inhibitors need to take them at the recommended dose in the recommended way. All protease inhibitors have a significant number of drug interactions. Therefore if someone is on a protease inhibitor, they must make sure that they are aware of these.

Retonavir is available in a capsule of 100mg strength. The normal dose is

600mg twice a day, therefore twelve capsules need to be taken daily. It is also available in a liquid form but this has a nasty taste and usually the capsules (which may be quite difficult to swallow) are preferred. When people start on Retonavir, because of the high incidence of side-effects, an escalating dose is recommended, for example, 300mg twice a day for three days, then 400mg twice a day for four days, 500mg twice a day for five days and finally the recommended dose of 600mg twice a day. It is advised that Retonavir is taken with food as this improves absorption. The drug has a limited life if not stored in a cool place, thus it is recommended that Retonavir is stored in a fridge (for up to 30 days) after it has been prescribed.

Common side-effects when starting Retonavir include nausea, vomiting, diarrhoea, tingling in the hands and feet and around the mouth, difficulty sleeping and very vivid dreams. Often people feel tired for some weeks after starting Retonavir. Most doctors prescribe Retonavir with an anti-diarrhoea agent and an anti-nausea tablet for the first few weeks. Some people manage Retonavir extremely well and experience very few side-effects, others have a more difficult time. Retonavir (like other protease inhibitors) interferes with glucose (sugar) metabolism and thus seems to increase blood sugars in people taking this medication. Latterly it has been found that some people develop a form of diabetes, which again is a significant side-effect. Retonavir and other protease inhibitors have also been found to interfere with blood cholesterol and triglyceride levels and hence doctors prescribing these drugs will continue to monitor patients closely.

Retonavir does have significant drug interactions. Any patient on Retonavir should have a full list of the drugs they should not take at the same time; these include diazepam (Valium), cisapride, terfenadine (Triludan), Co-proxamol, rifampicin and rifabutin. This is not a full list but it is very important that drugs that are contra-indicated with Retonavir are not taken at the same time.

Saquinavir (Invirase)

This is also a protease inhibitor that is taken in combination with other anti-virals and sometimes in combination with Retonavir itself. It is available in a capsule of 200mg strength. Its normal dose is 600mg three times a day but in use with Retonavir may be used at a dose of 400mg twice a day.

It is best to take Saquinavir with food and again it does have some significant drug interactions with other antibiotics (including Rifabutin and Rifampicin) and antihistamines (Triludan). Saquinavir commonly causes diarrhoea and abdominal pain when first starting. Other tablets may be given to reduce some of the side-effects. A new formulation of soft gel capsules is now available which is more effective.

Indinavir (Crixivan)

This is also a protease inhibitor. It is available in capsules at 200mg and 400mg strength and the normal dose is 800mg three times a day. It should be taken in doses at equally divided times and is also best taken either one hour before food or two hours after food. Ideally this food should be of a low-fat nature, in other words the food restrictions can be quite limiting. As a result of this some patients actively seek the advice of a dietician before embarking on Indinavir. Additionally it is important to drink at least one-and-a-half litres of liquid every day if a person is on Indinavir: one of the drug's side-effects is an increased risk of kidney stones that can be reduced by having a good fluid intake. Obviously in hot weather this fluid intake may need to be increased further. Again, Indinavir has significant drug interactions and should not be taken with rifabutin, rifampicin and some of the antihistamines. Common side-effects of Indinavir include nausea and vomiting, abdominal pain and tiredness.

Nelfinavir (Viracept)

This is a protease inhibitor that is not licensed in the UK although this is expected in the future. Nelfinavir comes in 250mg tablets and the best dose is unclear at the present time, but people are often prescribed 750mg three times a day. Nelfinavir is best taken with food as this increases absorption. Common side-effects include diarrhoea and abdominal pain, nausea and tiredness. Again it has significant drug interactions with such drugs as rifabutin, rifampicin, ketaconazole and some antihistamines.

DMP266

This is a new drug that shows promise for the future. It is given once a day and seems to have a good side-effect profile. It is available in clinical trials and on a 'compassionate release' basis only. The latter means that only people who cannot tolerate other drugs or who have used up all other treatment options can access the drug.

Taking anti-viral drugs: some guidelines

With all anti-virals it is extremely important that they are taken in the optimum way. Patients should be clear about what this is before embarking on a complex regime and ought to receive advice from their HIV doctors, pharmacist, and other clinicians. Some patients find that it is a good idea to practice taking a 'dummy run' of pills for a couple of weeks to make sure that they can fit a complex regime into their lifestyle. The real pills could be substituted by sweets so that patients could practise taking complex regimes around mealtimes, depending on what regime they are recommended.

The use of complex combinations of anti-virals has been given the abbreviated name of HAART or *Highly Active AntiRetroviral Therapy*. Newer trials have recently been published suggesting that three drugs in combination is more effective than two. However, it remains unclear which are the best three drugs to start with and this may be different in different patients.

It is a good idea not to take recreational drugs with these anti-virals, many of which are relatively new and their interactions are not fully known. Also street drugs are not pure and may be mixed up with lots of different drugs. Indeed there have been instances of people taking HIV medication (the protease inhibitors are a specific example) with 'ecstasy' tablets and suffering nasty consequences, including death. In addition, someone may be less likely to remember to take their anti-viral drugs regularly if they are taking recreational drugs.

As has been stated previously, resistance to anti-viral drugs, almost irrespective of the type of anti-viral medication, develops. This has implications for the person taking medication and also has implications for people that they may be having unprotected sex with. It is conceivable that such resistant forms of the virus could be passed on. In these newly infected people one might imagine that current treatments would be less effective. Therefore it is very important for anyone who is on anti-viral treatment to practise safe sex in the same way that it is important for any individual regardless of their HIV status.

These drugs are all extremely costly and in the current environment, there are limitations to how much the health budget can expand to incorporate these costly regimes. Patients can help by not stockpiling or wasting drugs. Most people may not realise that once a drug is prescribed, it cannot be re-used for someone else if it is returned to the pharmacy. Therefore hospitals are not keen to prescribe large numbers of these drugs and they should not be stockpiled, especially when they are first prescribed, in case people cannot tolerate them due to side-effects.

Drug trials

HIV is a new disease and new drugs are being developed all the time. Patients who are HIV-positive are often very willing to go on to drug trials, as this may be their best opportunity to access the newer and most effective drugs. When a patient is on a drug trial, they are very closely and carefully monitored by the doctors and research nurses in the hospital.

In some drug trials, 'placebo' drugs are used. A patient may be given a dummy sugar pill to see whether or not taking the 'active' drug is more or less effective than the placebo. People will be subdivided into two groups, one of whom will usually be receiving the placebo pill, and the other the actual drug on trial. Neither patient or doctor are aware whether or not the patient is actually receiving an active drug; this is to avoid bias in the trial and is called a 'double-blind' test. It is important to remember that consent is required for any trial, no matter how big or small.

Some patients are less willing to take part in a drug trial because of the uncertainty of outcome and effectiveness of the drug. No one should ever feel that they have been coerced or pushed into a drug trial. When a patient is on a trial it is made quite clear to them that they are able to stop taking that drug at any time in the future should they decide to do so.

Drug trials are very important ways of evaluating new drugs and without them it would be very difficult to judge which drugs are effective. It is only through drug trials that we have been able to establish that in HIV combinations of anti-viral drugs are more effective than taking one drug alone. This has only been recently discovered in a large trial conducted in both North America and in Europe (Delta Co-ordinating Committee 1996). These trials found that, especially in people who have not taken an anti-viral treatment in the past, taking at least two drugs (AZT and ddI or AZT and ddC) against HIV infection was much more effective than taking just one drug. The people that were in the group who took at least two drugs and had not been on any anti-viral treatment prior to this lived longer and suffered fewer HIV-related symptoms. Newer trials are now comparing two, three or four drugs.

Starting treatment

A variety of factors determine when to start treatment, most importantly the patient's wishes. Although there is no clear consensus about exactly when to start treatment, most doctors would agree that patients with persistent symptoms should be offered anti-viral treatment. However, many patients feel well but have immune tests that suggest their immune system is significantly damaged or that significant damage to the immune system is about to occur.

It seems that starting anti-viral treatment when the CD4 count is around about the 300 mark, or if it suddenly drops, is reasonable. The picture with viral load is less clear; however, most doctors would agree that anyone with a high viral load (over 100,000) should be offered treatment almost irrespective of their CD4 count. In people with viral loads of between 10,000 and 100,000, other factors need to be taken into account such as the patient's wishes, their CD4 count, the presence or absence of symptoms and previous blood results.

Switching treatment

Some patients are unable to tolerate some anti-viral drugs and need to be closely monitored because of side-effects. We know that the efficiency of drug combinations may not last indefinitely and that HIV is able to develop resistance to anti-viral treatments. When monitoring by CD4 count, viral load and symptoms indicates that resistance seems to be occurring, a new combination of treatment is advised. Most doctors would agree that changing all the anti-viral drugs previously used, if possible, is the best option. The situation currently is quite complicated as new drugs are available over a short space of time and many patients have a complex history of previous anti-viral treatment. Patients are also limited to which drugs are available in their particular hospital which, in turn, may depend upon factors such as which trials are ongoing and the cost of the medication. Overall this means the patient may be taking different combinations of different anti-viral drugs. Thus, switching therapies needs to be done on an individual basis, with discussions following immunological monitoring tests, taking into account patients' wishes, current medication and with 'an eye on' future drug options.

Drug treatments for AIDS-related illnesses

Many of the AIDS-related infections that people with HIV may develop can now be successfully treated with drugs. If someone is particularly unwell, these drugs need to be given intravenously, otherwise they can be given in tablet or liquid form. The table below shows what drugs are used to treat specific AIDS-related infections.

Other drug treatments

Below is a list of some commonly used drugs that are used to treat specific HIV-related symptoms:

1 Anti-diarrhoea medication includes Imodium, codeine phosphate and occasionally thalidomide.
2 Anti-depressants, including drugs such as Prozac and amitriptyline.
3 Appetite stimulants such as megestrol may be helpful for people with a poor appetite.

Table 8.1   Drug treatments for AIDS-related conditions

Drug	Drug use	Common side-effects	Common drug interactions and other information
Acyclovir (Zovirax)	Herpes infections	Occasionally nausea	
Amphotericin B	Fungal infections	Nausea, vomiting, fever, kidney failure	Given intravenously in hospital; close monitoring of kidney function needed
Atovaquone (Wellvone)	PCP and toxoplasmosis	Rash, nausea, diarrhoea	Take with a fatty meal
Bleomycin	KS	Fever, nausea, rarely lung damage	Given intravenously
Ciprofloxacin	MAI, antibiotic for infections	Rash, nausea, diarrhoea	Care if known allergy to penicillin
Clarithromycin (Klaricid)	MAI, antibiotic for infections	Nausea, abdominal pain	Take with food to reduce side-effects
Co-trimoxazole (Septrin)	PCP prevention and treatment	Rash, fever, headaches	Take with food to reduce side-effects
Fluconazole (Diflucan)	Thrush, prevention of recurrence of cryptococcal meningitis	Rash, nausea	
Foscarnet	CMV infections	Kidney damage, alteration in the blood levels of minerals, ulcers on the penis	Given intravenously usually, can be given as an injection in the eye
Ganciclovir (Cymevene)	CMV infections (eye, bowel)	Anaemia, nausea, headache	Can be given intravenously (stop other drugs which suppress the bone marrow); in tablet form take with food
Isoniazid	TB	Rash, liver damage, can damage nerve endings	Take on empty stomach
Itraconazole (Sporanox)	Thrush and other fungal infections	Nausea, rash	
Ketaconazole (Nizoral)	Fungal infections	Rash, nausea	Drug levels affected by some anti-virals; check with doctor
Liposomal Doxorubicin (Doxsil)	KS	Nausea, bone marrow suppression	Give intravenously
Pentamidine	PCP prevention and treatment	Cough, low blood sugar	Inhaled or intravenously (can cause kidney damage in intravenous form)
Pyrimethamine (Daraprim)	Toxoplasmosis	Bone marrow suppression, rash	
Rifabutin (Mycobutin)	MAI	Rash, nausea	Turns skin and body fluids reddish colour
Rifampicin (Rifadin)	TB	Rash, liver problems	Take on empty stomach
Vincristine/ Vinblastine	KS	Bone marrow suppression, hair loss, nausea, nerve damage	Give intravenously

4 Anti-nausea drugs. These are frequently given especially if someone is due to start on combination treatment of anti-virals as nausea is a common side-effect when initiating treatment. They may be given prophylactically. Commonly prescribed anti-nausea drugs include Maxolon, cyclizine, haloperidol and ondansetron.

This is not an exhaustive list of all the treatments that someone with HIV-related symptoms may take. Information should be provided by the doctor prescribing medication and the dispensing pharmacy. It is important to remember that drugs may have significant drug interactions especially with the newer protease inhibitors. Therefore it is important to clarify whether any new medication prescribed, even if it is over-the-counter (OTC) medication, can be taken safely with the HIV medication.

People with HIV infection can be safely vaccinated should they wish to travel to countries where vaccinations are recommended. Children with HIV infection should be vaccinated also. The only potential problem with vaccinations and HIV infection is in the case of live vaccines. There are few live vaccines (oral polio, yellow fever and BCG) and in some of these cases, for example polio, alternative killed vaccinations are available.

If someone with HIV infection is travelling to malarial areas they should take anti-malaria prophylaxis as recommended. It is worth also saying that certain groups of people with HIV infection such as gay men and injecting drug-users may be at greater risk of hepatitis B infection. There is a safe and effective vaccine that can be given against this. Interestingly, in the immediate few weeks post-vaccination, a viral load test may be transiently elevated because of stimulation to the immune system. There is no evidence that vaccinations cause any progression of HIV infection.

Drug treatments in patients with advanced HIV disease

Drug regimes can become increasingly complex as people develop advanced HIV disease. Some of the issues raised are dealt with in Chapters 4 and 11. However, if someone is on complex medication a 'dosset box' may be very helpful to sub-divide drug treatments. Community nurse specialists may help with arranging to obtain one of these. Dosset boxes are small boxes where medication is divided into appropriate sections to be taken throughout the day. This means that the drugs are easier to remember to take and carers can check to see whether medication has been taken.

Syringe drivers are sometimes used when people have intractable symptoms and are unable to control these symptoms by taking tablets orally. A syringe driver is a small syringe which is attached to a box. The syringe has a needle with a small lead attached to it that is placed under the skin, usually on the abdominal wall. The box can then be kept in a pocket. Through this mechanism drugs can be delivered on a 24-hour basis as a continual infusion. Often this is a good way to try and control pain or nausea that may be common in people with advanced HIV infection. Once the symptoms are under control, the syringe driver may be swapped for tablets again.

Complementary medicines

Many people with HIV infection will investigate alternative and complementary medicines. There is an enormous range of these therapies available, including homeopathy, Chinese herbal medicine and acupuncture. We do not intend to go in to these therapies in any specific detail. It is worth saying however that they can be very beneficial and are unlikely to do harm. However, it is worth going to a reputable practitioner as, unfortunately, the boom in complementary medicines has meant that there are some less reputable people making money out of therapies which are largely unproven. It is always important to tell any doctors that one may be seeing exactly what alternative therapies one is taking. There have been documented cases of complications following the use of alternative medicines. Most of these therapies are not available on the NHS and it may be worth shopping around also to make sure that one is getting value for money!

Further information regarding anti-retrovirals can also be obtained from the CRUSAID-STAR Information Exchange, 369 Fulham Road, London SW10 9NH.

References

Bartlett, J. (1996) 'Protease Inhibitors for HIV Infection', *Annals of Internal Medicine*, 124: 1086–8.
Carpenter, C., Fischl, M., Hammer, S. et al. (1996) 'Consensus statement – Antiretroviral Therapy for HIV Infection 1996: Recommendations of an International Panel', *Journal of the American Medical Association*, 276: 146–56.
Delta Co-ordinating Committee (1996), 'Delta: a randomised double blind controlled trial comparing combinations of zidovudine plus didanosine or zalcitabine with zidovudine alone in HIV infected individuals', *Lancet*, 348: 283–91.

9 Change, Uncertainty and Complex Issues in HIV and AIDS

'Change, we must remember, with all its difficulties, is inescapable' (Benedict 1935, p. 26)

This chapter aims to integrate key messages from previous chapters under three main themes. Using two case histories several quite complex issues are described and explored. One of these themes – that of change – is predominant because it is characteristic of this field of medicine. Moreover, one recurrent message about HIV infection and AIDS should now be clear and that is simply the fact that it has social and psychological consequences which are sometimes hard to define and even more difficult to resolve.

This chapter contains information about such topics as antenatal HIV testing and the uncertainty of long-term anti-retroviral therapy. These are just two factors that indicate why clinical management and policy regarding aspects of ante-natal care, in both hospitals and the community, will continue to evolve as new information comes to light.

These three topics – change, complexity and the need to deal with uncertainty – form the basis of this chapter. They will be described in three sections:

1 Should there be more widespread antenatal HIV testing in the United Kingdom?
2 Complex issues in families infected with and affected by HIV infection.
3 Transitional states and treatment in HIV infection and AIDS.

Should there be more widespread antenatal HIV testing in the United Kingdom?

Even though in the United Kingdom (UK) the current epidemic of HIV has thankfully not reached predicted proportions, a significant number of people infected with HIV remain undetected. This factor alone probably means that in the near future there will be more widespread offering of HIV testing, particularly of women thinking of having children and those in the early stages of pregnancy. While this strategy appears to target women as if it was their sole burden, there are cogent reasons why a new initiative would undoubtedly be beneficial to mothers and their children. The main reasons are as follows.

Anonymous antenatal screening (see Chapter 1), where HIV tests are carried out in a variety of clinical settings but *cannot* be traced back to the patient, suggests that 87 per cent of women who are HIV-positive in London and the South-east are unaware of their HIV status (DOH 1996). Other studies also suggest that often these same patients present to a range of health care services (for example general practitioners and hospital clinics) even though up until then they have not been diagnosed with HIV infection (Madge et al. 1997). The net effect of these findings is that since the early 1980s, approximately 300 babies have been born with HIV infection or AIDS in the UK each year. In the majority of cases the diagnosis will have been made after the birth of the baby. Indeed, some babies are so unwell that they are diagnosed with AIDS and this is the first indication that they are HIV-positive (Noone et al. 1997, PHLS 1997).

This problem is preventable in the new-born: if women can be identified prior to, or even at the time of pregnancy, the options for the mother are naturally greater. Of course, it may not be possible to reduce overall morbidity (overall suffering) to nothing, however giving either the mother or the parents the choice in such difficult circumstances will undoubtedly prove beneficial for all concerned. Moreover, if the infection is diagnosed early, the greatest benefits may be seen in the newborn child where specialised monitoring and treatments can now be used to substantial effect. The specific interventions are highlighted below.

First, the use of certain anti-retroviral medications such as Zidovudine (AZT) in the ante-natal period and possible delivery by Caesarian section are proven to reduce the chances of the child acquiring the infection perinatally (DOH 1996). Second, there is good evidence that transmission of the virus to the child (called vertical transmission) can be substantially reduced by not breast-feeding the new-born baby (see Chapter 2). The virus can be isolated from all body fluids and breast milk is no different from any other bodily fluid (see Chapters 1–3).

As a result there needs to be a frank discussion between patient and clinician in these circumstances. Often the patient's general practitioner is a valued source of objective advice and guidance. Hospital and community clinics are becoming adept at presenting information such as this in culturally sensitive, patient-friendly ways. However, where this is not available, other organisations in the area such as special interest groups or Community Health Councils (CHC) may be able to help.

Some may ask – quite appropriately – why there has not been a louder, clearer, even earlier call for such testing in the light of the information presented above. Despite Department of Health guidelines, the uptake for HIV testing (that is, those people who agree to be tested when offered) in hospital and community antenatal clinics has been remarkably low, even in London where HIV prevalence is highest (Chrystie et al. 1995, DOH 1996). Thus the detection rates of women with HIV infection remain low, even in areas of highest prevalence in the UK. This is in stark contrast to other European countries such as France where there is a detection rate of over 90 per cent of all HIV-infected babies.

Worryingly, in the UK, it is the high-prevalence, urban areas which merit extra attention. In such areas – which are not restricted to London boroughs – HIV infection and other sexually transmitted diseases are often associated with poverty, ethnicity and other socio-economic factors (Lacey et al. 1997). And, as has been pointed out before, there are other infections which are more insidious and less emotive but which can result in much distress. In other words, it is in these areas where needs are greatest and where resources, including the availability of high-quality clinicians such as doctors and nurses are often most lacking. The reasons why there has not been much success in increasing the number of tests in antenatal clinics are complex. Actual testing for HIV in patients is undoubtedly one factor although the overall philosophy about HIV testing has changed significantly over the last ten years (see Chapter 2).

Initially, there was an understandable reluctance on the part of doctors, general practitioners in particular, to test for HIV infection except when it was 'clinically indicated'. In other words in the recent past, the overall thinking was not to look too hard for HIV infection, perhaps on the basis that nothing could be done anyway. Latterly, much more is known about HIV infection and its various manifestations. Furthermore many opportunistic infections can now be prevented and certainly identified earlier, which means that treatment is more effective. Lastly, the appearance of combination anti-retroviral therapies has resulted in a cautious optimism regarding HIV infection.

Part of this process is that clinicians, including general practitioners, are becoming more used to testing for HIV infection. Thus amongst clinicians, the need to 'normalise' the HIV test is becoming more common, especially in high-prevalence areas. Hence, a rather more pragmatic approach is being advocated where a number of the issues surrounding an HIV test can be discussed just like other more routine blood tests (DOH 1994).

One of reasons why this type of testing may lend itself to community and general practice settings is that GPs and practice nurses are traditionally very familiar with their practice population. Moreover this strategy is entirely consistent with the current guidance from the Department of Health which favours a 'discussion' around the test and not 'counselling' (DOH 1996). The scope for HIV prevention within a wider sexual health promotion is rightfully seen to be part of primary care. In addition, the relaxation of insurer's guidelines with respect to negative HIV tests and heightened awareness of HIV infection may mean that more patients are willing to discuss and request HIV testing in primary care (see Chapters 2 and 6).

Chronic HIV infection and AIDS impact on individuals, families and children and the general public ought to be able to expect certain standards of care from their general practitioner and the wider primary care team. To deny this is to deny the progress made in HIV and AIDS care.

As noted above, being able to present this information to women in user-friendly, culturally sensitive ways may be 'half the battle'. It would be wrong, inappropriate and crass to assume that all women know about and understand these complex issues. One of the greatest challenges is to translate this information into individually-tailored packages which can then be modified for women who have their own special needs, for example women with a limited understanding of such issues, teenagers and adolescents and women from ethnic minorities. The latter group particularly need information which is presented in culturally-friendly ways. Lastly, it would be wrong if initiatives such as these were perceived to be targeting foreign nationals. It is a fine line between 'targeting' information and 'scape-goating' certain groups (see next page).

One last point needs a mention. The ethical stance of *not* identifying women and children at the earliest stages is dubious in view of the prevailing evidence and the current availability of resources. Clinicians work within the best limits of the evidence wherever possible and this is an area where the evidence is becoming more compelling. Preventable morbidity and mortality of HIV-related antenatal and perinatal conditions requires a more effective way of identifying early HIV infection and AIDS; this probably means a more determined effort to test more women in the early ante-natal period.

Case history

J. is a 32-year-old Zairian refugee who has been in the UK for the last 18 months. She is pregnant. Her husband M., aged 37, is supportive and they are both seeking asylum in the UK on political grounds. They live in North London.

She presented to her general practitioner when she was around six months pregnant. At the booking appointment in hospital, J., accompanied by her husband, is offered HIV testing because it is the policy of the particular unit to offer it to all expectant mothers. The majority of the discussion is completed by the midwife on the unit. J. consents to the test, fully expecting that the result will return as negative. Thus blood tests are taken for all the routine antenatal tests including rubella, syphilis serology and antibodies to HIV infection. Both husband and wife are in good health and neither have any 'medical' worries. Neither are especially concerned about HIV infection, although they both had friends who were HIV-positive in Zaire.

The test results return: J. is found to be HIV-positive. J. is again accompanied by her husband and the midwife breaks the news gently and tactfully. The immediate plan is to refer J. to the medical team in the same teaching hospital, while continuing to ensure she is seen regularly by the specialist HIV midwife.

Initially, J. is very shocked by the result. She has more blood taken from her for a confirmatory result and also her CD4 count is measured along with the newer tests of viral load. These results return as showing a CD4 count of 370 and a viral load of 7000 copies/ml. These show that she is moderately immune-compromised, although she has a relatively low viral load.

Over the ensuing week a number of issues are discussed with J. including the main priority, about which she is agreed, of how to minimise vertical transmission to her unborn child. Meanwhile, her husband, M. has also been thinking about the implications these results have for himself. While at the moment his main concern is the welfare of his wife and unborn child, he knows that perhaps soon he may want to find out his own HIV status.

After two weeks and a number of discussions with many clinicians and professionals, she agrees to commence AZT (Zidovudine). Despite being keen to breast-feed her baby, she now knows that this would be risky to her newborn child. She remains, understandably, very ambivalent about this and may well not agree to this aspect of her baby's care. She has, however, agreed to an elective Caesarian section for the delivery of the child, because of the higher risk of transmitting the virus in the normal labouring process.

J. is therefore admitted to the labour ward at about 38 weeks gestation and a baby girl, birth weight 7lbs, is delivered by Caesarian section. The newborn is bottle-fed, her mother having changed her mind almost at the last moment.

As can be seen from the case history, patients with chronic HIV infection and AIDS have to cope with a disease which is serious and distressing and also affects ordinary social customs and beliefs. The added problem of HIV infection and AIDS as stigmatising only compounds the distress for those affected. This stigma can also affect family members or members of the informal social network. In the case of J. and M. and their unborn child, there are other complex issues which inevitably come to the fore, for example what about J.'s husband and his status? What will all this mean for their future relationship? Who else ought to know about J.'s new HIV status?

Adjusting to HIV infection

It is accepted that people adjust, or more accurately re-adjust to a diagnosis of HIV infection in a variety of ways. The most important point is that a degree of adjustment is both inevitable and necessary in order for 'life to go on'. It is common for three characteristics – shock, anger and denial – to be prominent amongst the first reactions.

Shock

While some people adjust very rapidly to this devastating news, others take much longer. One of the factors which may influence this process is how expected was the diagnosis at the time of testing. Intuitively a person half-expecting to be told they are HIV-positive will already be some way to accepting this is now part of their life. For someone else who is not expecting to be told they are HIV-positive (for example, J. in the case history), perhaps because of a single sexual encounter, the news can be a tremendous shock and leave the person feeling numbed, distressed and traumatised.

In the last case it was exceedingly difficult to broach the subject of causality and some may argue for little gain. What was known was that J.

had tested positive and that a significant adjustment period would be necessary if she (and all her family) were to adapt to this condition.

In these circumstances much depends on how the health professional – usually a doctor – has handled giving this bad news. This task, the one of 'handling bad news' has major training implications for health care professionals. It is now common for clinicians of all types, doctors included, to be offered training in 'giving and handling bad news' within a context of enhancing their communication skills. In many ways this type of training is no different to learning how to complete a surgical procedure. If training has not been undertaken, there is a good chance that this aspect of care will be deficient.

Anger

It is often the case that someone given an HIV diagnosis will suffer mood swings, perhaps as part of the 'anger' which can be a feature of this early phase. This feature may well depend on how they have coped with stresses in a general way. It is also very easy to underestimate this anger or rage at this point in time. These feelings may be due to several interrelated factors, of which HIV infection is one. For example, coping with the stigma of using injectable drugs or, having to tell family members of the diagnosis may be particular stress factors in a person's life, which are also contributing to the anger at a particular moment in time.

For some, it may be the culmination of a series of life-events, starting off from being abused in childhood, to leaving home, and ending up with HIV infection. The point is that there are many reasons for anger and focusing entirely on HIV infection may not be appropriate for the person concerned. One strategy is to continue with a set routine for a few days, although this is always easier said than done. The initial shock will, with time, subside; however, as stated previously, this will depend on a number of factors. One easy way of doing this is to ensure that the person affected continues to work (if they are working anyway). Nevertheless, for others, this may be impossible and thus a time for thoughtful reflection may be in order.

Denial

Denial is a phase that is perhaps the most difficult, though for the person concerned they may appear totally oblivious to this. It is sometimes easy to regard denial as a wholly negative notion and one which either hinders or certainly does not help the healing process. This is a fairly negative way of viewing what is really everybody's mechanism for 'putting off until tomorrow what cannot be done today'. In other words, it is a normal part of life that people with painful or difficult experiences are able to deal with such delicate matters at a more appropriate time. Denial in terms of HIV infection and AIDS is no different, although it may be frustrating for those closest to the person with the newly diagnosed HIV infection.

Perhaps at the beginning a person may deny they have HIV infection, even though they know, however this is usually time-limited. (This is another reason why safe sex is imperative since people may not, almost unknowingly, admit to being HIV-positive.) Individuals vary in their 'use' of this natural mechanism of denial and it is common for those to use it at judicious moments though these may all occur subconsciously. Denial may be a feature of early diagnosis, but then also at various times later on. For example, there may be elements of denial at the time of first symptoms, or perhaps at the first serious opportunistic infection or at the time that the CD4 cells start to diminish.

It is also important to note that these stages of adjustment are not fixed and well-delineated. No aspect of human behaviour can ever be described as so, though some would like to think so. This description of shock, anger and denial owes much to Elizabeth Kubler-Ross in the context of dying. She described a Western, individual-oriented approach to very painful experiences exemplified by 'death and dying' (Kubler-Ross 1970). It is now accepted that these features overlap, merge and coincide in a way that was not fully appreciated previously. Thus a person may be angry, almost to the point of rage, but these episodes alternate distressingly with periods of denial where concerns about HIV infection and AIDS are submerged for a few days or weeks. It is thus pragmatic to view these concepts – shock, anger, denial – as oscillating and overlapping. The various components can be described as a process through which people traverse in a way which is highly individual and personal, as arguably it ought to be. Any attempt to constrain this process can be seen to be 'psychologising' a normal reaction to stressful events.

Complex issues in families infected and affected with HIV infection

The main purpose for highlighting the case history below, which is based upon a true narrative, is to illustrate a number of key issues: it identifies the importance of the roles of different professionals; it explains how boundaries between patient and professional are sometimes a basic requirement which protects both patient and clinician alike, and finally, it highlights how effective communication between all of those caring for families can pay dividends.

Similar to the previous case, there is the possibility of more than one member of the family having chronic HIV infection. For health care professionals, such cases may appear overwhelming.

Case history

Q. is a 33-year-old Ugandan refugee who lives in London. She has lived in London for the past three years. She escaped from her own country during a time of political turmoil. During this escape she was separated from her children, Janet, aged 11 and Eva, aged 3, but later they were thankfully reunited. Latterly, during her time in Uganda, she experienced much persecution and was imprisoned for a short while. She also witnessed executions. She knows that many of her family members were killed and does not know the whereabouts of others. During her time in prison she was raped.

Here in the UK, she does not work, and she is in receipt of benefits. She first presented to her general practitioner (GP) with a cough, tiredness, night-sweats and weight loss. Her GP was also concerned about Q.'s youngest child, Eva, who had persistent lymph node swellings in her neck and bilateral parotitis (inflammation and swelling of the parotid gland in both her cheeks). The GP had raised HIV testing with Q. on several occasions, particularly in relation to Eva; however, Q. had declined. As Q. herself became increasingly unwell, she was admitted to hospital. After investigations she was found to have tuberculosis (TB) and as a result, it was important for the clinicians to exclude HIV infection. An HIV test was again recommended to Q. and she accepted.

She was found to be HIV-positive, which was subsequently confirmed with further tests. Q. was very distressed by this news, since she was hoping that she had somehow escaped this one last assault on her. She had had episodes of depression in the past and found this news almost too much to bear. She was provided with support and medical follow-up on discharge and she responded well to her anti-TB treatment. Unfortunately she remained resistant to taking any other HIV therapies because she firmly believed they would not help her.

After several months it became apparent that Eva was becoming increasingly unwell. After much discussion, Q. agreed that both Eva and Janet should have HIV tests. Eva's test was found to be positive and Janet's was negative. Obviously Q. was relieved at Janet's result but found the confirmation of Eva's HIV-positive status extremely traumatic and distressing. Eva was seen by a paediatrician at the same hospital unit and followed up thereafter.

Because of all of these events and circumstances, Q. remains depressed. Her stage of HIV disease remains precarious and she is resistant to taking any conventional HIV therapies, choosing to wait 'until she becomes ill'. She does, however, attend for regular follow-up and has good links with a dietitian, her general practitioner and practice-based counsellor and community nurse specialists. Eva's HIV status remains stable. She has not become unwell on account of the HIV infection and thus, there is no indication for further therapy such as anti-retroviral therapy.

Janet, who is now approaching twelve years, has begun to ask questions as to why her mother and sister need so many visits to the hospital. Q. has agonized as to whether or not she should tell Janet the truth of their HIV status.

This case has been somewhat simplified! However, many complex issues and equally complex dilemmas arise from the history, some of which are illustrated below. It is perhaps the combination of such difficult circumstances, the lack of overall guidance and the pragmatic nature of Q.'s attitude which makes the case so challenging.

Physical

Q.'s increasing ill-health is, of course, a major concern not only to herself but also to those looking after her. It is clear that already she has had a serious co-infection with HIV, that is, tuberculosis. In addition, Q. suffers with depression, perhaps as a result of these various episodes of ill-health, although there are many other reasons, including her recent past. She also finds caring for her two children difficult at times, especially since she has little support at hand.

Although a number of clinicians have discussed other therapies, for example anti-retroviral medications, Q. is fairly determined that she should not have these at the moment. Certainly several clinicians hope that with gentle encouragement Q. will agree to starting anti-retroviral therapy in the not too distant future.

Psychological

The whole issue of what and when to tell which of the children about the HIV diagnoses is extremely complex and needs preparation and expert advice. Q.'s depression is a compounding factor and one which hinders her genuine attempts to properly care for her children. Her depression is not altogether surprising given her past history of multiple bereavements and trauma in her country of origin. Janet, the eldest of the two daughters, is likely to continue to be suspicious about her mother's and sister's ill-health but will need support when she finds out the truth.

Q. has had several courses of anti-depressants although she does not like 'the tablets' because they make her tired and sleepy. Moreover these tablets (anti-depressants) cause headaches and she suffers with a dry mouth while taking them.

Cultural

It is likely that even if Q. had not been found to be HIV-positive that she may have found adapting to a new culture difficult. She has little support in this country and she has no partner, family or close friends. The benefit, housing and social security system can be extremely perplexing for someone who is from this country and culture but may be quite overwhelming for someone who isn't.

Perhaps more importantly for Q. is how she regards HIV infection in the more general sense. For example, she has had friends with HIV infection in Africa. The various meanings attached in Africa to this rampant infection may well be very different from those in the West. Certainly, treatment issues will be completely different, since very little anti-retroviral therapy is generally available in many African countries.

Generally, beliefs and perceptions play a critical role in how people (of all cultural groups) make decisions about if and when to accept treatment. For example, in order to try and explore how Q. feels towards these newer medications it is necessary to find out the extent of her knowledge. Her perceptions about the role of the medication, how long it is to be taken for, what sort of side-effects it will have, and the possible effect on her children, will feature highly in her concerns about this type of medication. Ultimately, it will govern whether she takes it as recommended or not (see p. 148).

With these concerns in mind, Q. was asked what her current list of problems were and she prioritised the following list herself:

- Her HIV status
- Her daughter's HIV status
- Her own and her daughter's physical health and mental health
- The future of her daughter Janet
- The future of both her children should she die first
- Her refugee status in this country
- Her housing
- Her current income
- Concerns about her family back home
- Coping with trauma suffered in the years prior to leaving her country (witnessing executions and other brutalities including her rape).

It is easy to assume that HIV is the problem that Q. would put at the top of her list. However, frequently other more mundane but equally distressing problems such as income, housing, children's health, refugee status are as likely to be important.

Practical

A large number of people are involved in this case, including the hospital doctors, the dietician, hospital counsellors, community nurse specialist and general practitioner. The reasons for good communication are obvious as are role definitions and maintaining boundaries.

Transitional states and treatment in HIV infection and AIDS

Several stages of HIV infection can be delineated which have psycho-emotional implications for those with HIV infection. The transition from HIV infection to symptomatic disease and from the latter to AIDS are two of these critical phases.

Symptomatic disease

Adjustment to increasing but relatively minor infections may be difficult, especially if previously the individual has been healthy. For the patient this may represent the obvious decline towards the development of more serious illnesses and even AIDS. While this belief, perhaps even expectation, is not unreasonable, it ultimately depends on other parameters (for example other investigations) as to whether a period of deterioration is imminent or not. In many cases, this is just impossible to predict – an aspect that people affected, carers and family members as well as clinicians find wildly frustrating. Once again it is prudent to note that people with HIV infection and AIDS can also suffer with non-HIV related complaints and often reassurance about this is needed.

AIDS

The first AIDS diagnosis may occur many years after the HIV diagnosis. Previously and much more commonly individuals acquired an AIDS diagnosis at the same time as their HIV diagnosis. Clearly simultaneous HIV and AIDS diagnoses are inevitably more serious and are quite distressing to all concerned. In this case the many issues related to this new diagnosis are focused in a way that can cause great anxiety in those affected.

A diagnosis of AIDS again represents a watershed in the natural history – arguably the natural progression – of chronic HIV infection. Among the important issues that emerge at this time is the need for extra visits to the hospital, perhaps leading to a greater dependency on doctors and nurses. Other prominent issues include impending ill-health, the loss of control this may entail and perhaps a realisation, for the very first time, that personal mortality is inevitable.

Information about HIV and AIDS monitoring

The fact that HIV/AIDS monitoring has recently changed to incorporate new aspects such as 'viral load' signifies that little in HIV and AIDS information is static for long. Viral load is a relatively new monitoring tool which allows a more accurate assessment of how much active human immune-deficiency virus is in circulation through the body (see Chapter 3). It is traditionally measured in terms of 'copies' of HIV RNA per millilitre (copies/ml) (NAM Aug 97).

Clinically and statistically, individuals with high viral loads are more likely to develop the complications of chronic HIV infection than those with low counts. However, importantly – and this is common to managing many conditions in medicine – no single test can ever predict how a particular individual will fare in the future. Thus it is inappropriate and generally medically unsound to identify a person's viral load as exclusively indicative of deciding 'how long they are going to live'. Nothing in medicine works like that.

Starting treatment

The prevailing trend is for people to commence treatment much sooner than in previous times. Starting anti-retroviral treatment (see below), however is a highly significant step along what can be a capricious path. Why is this the case?

First, once treatment is started, there is really an implicit commitment that treatment is continuous for the foreseeable future. In other words, once on this treatment there is no coming off, although there are *always* exceptions. While this may mean a particular stage has been reached in the natural history of HIV, commencing treatment can also present certain practical problems such as remembering to take the medicine on a daily basis. This is why it is absolutely essential that this decision is not taken lightly. Patients are right to discuss such decisions with a number of different clinicians such as the clinic nurse or doctor. It is also common for individuals to obtain so-called independent advice, something which is to be encouraged. The patient's general practitioner can be a good source of this independent advice.

Second, the medication regimes which use a combination of therapies and which appear to be successful – although long-term studies do not exist as yet for obvious reasons – require major effort on the patient's part. While some need to be taken with food, others require an empty stomach. Often particular foods should be avoided, and of course, the potential drug interactions with more standard medications (for example antibiotics) need to be carefully monitored (see Chapter 8 for details). To reiterate a previous point, the decision to commence anti-retroviral therapy ought to be a considered one, especially taking into account the various implications of the therapy.

Third, the exact timing of the more aggressive therapies, sometimes called combination or HAART (Highly Active Anti-Retroviral Therapy) appears crucial but is as yet unknown. Many think that, in order for such drugs to be effective, they ought to be administered early in the course of the infection. The idea of such therapy is to reduce the viral load, that is, the amount of active virus in the body, to almost nothing, or certainly to undetectable levels. However, other more conservative clinicians feel that there is only 'one bite to this cherry' and to use this up early in the course of the infection may, in the long run, not be in the best interests of the patient. This is especially important when taking into account that better prevention and earlier recognition of complications has already increased survival for those with HIV infection and AIDS without the use of such drugs.

As stated above, the long-term side-effects of such medications cannot be fully known simply because they have not been around long enough.

Nevertheless, this is also another important factor in trying to weigh up the benefits and drawbacks in making an informed decision about HAART.

Fourth, and related to the above, it may well be that, although these new medications appear to be more effective, they will have a time-limited effect on HIV. The main reason for this is viral resistance to the new therapies (Greener 1997). Perhaps more worrying is that, because HIV is known to have a very high mutation rate, resistance to one particular drug may protect the virus from other anti-viral therapies. In other words once resistance appears, changing medications may well only marginally improve matters since the virus will have acquired resistance to these other newer ones (this is called 'cross-resistance'). Although resistance is a common occurrence in microbiology, it seems that this factor is the reason why HAART will almost certainly be time-limited.

Finally, whether HAART will really be able to eradicate HIV infection totally or simply suppress its effects for a finite time remains, as yet, unknown. In the latter case, where suppression is maximal, there is less chance of resistance to the virus.

What is important is that this pattern of drug development, fast-tracking of its production and its introduction into clinical trials has been seen before with Zidovudine, the first anti-retroviral medication on the market. In this latter case, the effectiveness of Zidovudine was shown to be time-limited and it is not inconceivable that this pattern is being repeated with the new HAART therapies. Only time will tell. Whether this pattern is endlessly repeating – the details may well be different with the use of single, double, triple or even quadruple therapy – remains undetermined at this stage.

'Compliance'

Until recently, the term 'compliance' was thought about in terms of whether patients were taking their medications. While this is still the case, there is a move towards 'concordance', because the latter term seems to underline a more equitable power relationship between patient and doctor (Mullen 1997). The reason why 'compliance' or 'concordance' (the exact term is really not relevant) is even more critical in the field of HIV/AIDS treatment is that, theoretically, where medications are taken erratically or only intermittently, there is a greater chance that the virus will be able to build up a resistance.

Potential virus resistance is one reason why so much effort is made to provide as much information as possible to people who are about to embark on this type of multiple therapy, indeed so much so, that in parts of the country, doctors, pharmacists and nurse-practitioners have established 'compliance-clinics' in order to ensure the drugs are maximally effective (see Chapter 7). While this is important, it may reflect a relative lack of information which was provided in the past. 'Non-compliance' occurs for particular reasons, often because people perceive the medications are affecting them in unforseen ways. This is why, as suggested above, that the decision to embark on therapy is taken after due consideration, preferably after discussing it with various people including experts, family, friends and partner.

A recent publication suggests 'twenty questions' ought to be asked at the time of considering any medication (TAT 1996). These questions may be legitimately asked of any medication irrespective of the HIV status of the person, for example:

- What is the name of the drug?
- What does it look like?
- How and when should it be taken?
- How is it going to help?
- What if I feel ill on it?
- Can I drink alcohol with it?
- Should I take it on an empty or full stomach?
- Is it safe to drive while taking it?

Keeping up-to-date?

Not everybody chooses to keep themselves up-to-date with the various drug developments in the field of HIV and AIDS. Many people, like those with other medical conditions, are perfectly pleased to delegate this responsibility to a professional, such as a clinician. While it is common for some people to refer to publications like the National AIDS Manual (NAM), orthodox medical journals, and Internet websites, others are content to leave this to the clinical experts.

When the media is used as a source of new information, great caution needs to be exercised since misrepresentation is all too common. Often media stories headlined by 'HIV and AIDS: cure soon' completely distort genuine breakthroughs in monitoring and treatment of various aspects of these conditions. Of course to people affected, their partners and families, these stories can be frustrating and distressing.

Conclusion

The advent of combination therapies, known as the acronym HAART, has clearly brought with it a degree of cautious optimism. This optimism must be tempered with a number of problems, such as drug-resistance and the sheer daily effort in taking multiple drugs in order to achieve maximal suppression of human immuno-deficiency virus. As has been described, the long-term effects of these newer medications remain unknown.

While this description is necessarily scientific, it is easy to forget the human person who is faced with these decisions and the medicine. How someone takes their medication is critical both to themselves and more generally, especially if taken erratically.

The person taking the medicine must be party to discussions about the various components of drug therapy. And of course, no decision is ever irrevocable, although in this case, it is clearly not a good idea to oscillate between taking and not taking them. In such a circumstance it is better to not commence treatment and to consider carefully again the advantages and disadvantages about starting treatment.

References

Benedict, Ruth (1935) *Patterns of Culture*, London: Routledge & Kegan Paul.

Chrystie, I.L., Wolfe, C.D.A., Kennedy, J. et al. (1995) 'Voluntary testing for HIV in a community based antenatal clinic: a pilot study', *British Medical Journal*, 311: 928–31.

(DOH) Department of Health (1994) 'Guidelines for offering voluntary named HIV antibody-testing to women receiving ante-natal care', London: Department of Health.

(DOH) Department of Health (1996) 'Guidelines for pre-test discussion on HIV-testing 1996', London: Department of Health.

Greener, M. (1997) 'HIV resistance: The Achilles heel of AIDS treatment', *The AIDS letter: The Royal Society of Medicine*, No. 62, Aug./Sept.

Kubler-Ross, E. (1970) *On death and dying*, London: Tavistock Publications.

Lacey, C.J.N., Merrick, D.W., Bensley, D. et al. (1997) 'Analysis of the socio-demography of gonorrhoea in Leeds 1989–93'. *British Medical Journal*, 314: 1715–18.

Madge, S., Olaitan, A., Morcroft, A., Phillips, A.N. and Johnson, M.A. (1997) 'Access to medical care one year prior to diagnosis in one hundred HIV positive women', *Family Practice*, 14: 255–7.

Mullen, P.D. (1997) 'Compliance becomes Concordance', *British Medical Journal*, 314: 691–20.

NAM (1997) *National AIDS Manual/AIDS directory: a directory of a range of services*, London: NAM Publications.

Noone, A. and Goldberg, D. (1997) 'Antenatal testing: what now', *British Medical Journal*, 314: 1429–30.

PHLS (Public Health Laboratory Service) (1997) *Unlinked anonymous HIV prevalence monitoring programme: England and Wales survey of antenatal clinic attenders – results to December 1996*, London: PHLS.

TAT (Treatment Task Force) (1996) 'Minimum standards of care (for adults with HIV)', Leaflet produced by Lithosphere, London.

10 Palliative Care of People with HIV and AIDS

Introduction

While it is common for most clinicians in general to regard HIV infection and AIDS as a chronic condition, there is little doubt that it still has a variable though poor prognosis. Since the start of the epidemic 10,000 people have died in the UK from AIDS. It is therefore sensible to discuss palliative care issues in the context of planning services to individual patients.

Palliative care is formally defined as 'that stage of any condition where, following an accurate diagnosis, the advent of death is certain and not too far distant and for whom treatment has changed from the curative to the palliative' (OHE 1991).

This chapter deals specifically with the management of pain and several other common symptoms seen in the advanced stages of disease. In effect it looks at similar issues as those in Chapter 4, though in more detail. In keeping with planning and forethought, a number of points are made about living wills and advanced directives. While these documents are necessarily formal, they point the way to a more rigorous statement of a person's wishes towards the end of their life. Nowhere is this more salient than in the arena of HIV infection and AIDS.

It is necessary to acknowledge that in the developing countries the problems are entirely different and invariably worse. In many parts of the world, a diagnosis of HIV infection is tantamount to a terminal illness, and a fairly short one at that. The new optimism in HIV care cannot be shared due to resource issues, rampant co-infections such as tuberculosis and lack of palliative care teams. In such circumstances clinicians can do little except, where resources allow, point the way to care which aims to ameliorate symptoms.

It is important from the outset to acknowledge that, for the time being, many of the questions surrounding HIV infection and AIDS will remain unanswered, for a number of reasons. Quite simply, the human immuno-deficiency virus was only isolated at the beginning of the 1980s, although its existence had been proven before then (see Chapters 1 and 2). The Acquired Immune Deficiency Syndrome is a collection of disease entities, arbitrarily defined in the US and in Europe, which is thought to result from a declining immune system secondary to HIV infection. Thus, human immuno-deficiency virus and AIDS-related conditions have not been around long enough for all questions about pathophysiology and immunology to be clarified and resolved.

While a whole range of advances have been made in the interrelated fields of microbiology, virology, immunology and clinical medicine in general, much work remains before definitive answers will be possible. For example, many people talk about the possibility of a vaccine; however, the virus mutates at such a rate that a vaccine appears to be a distant hope rather than an immediate reality.

Although the approach in this text is fairly cautious, there is evidence that a breakthrough is occurring and is regarded with real and genuine hope amongst those affected by HIV infection and AIDS. The advent of combination therapies and newer, more sophisticated monitoring methods for those with HIV infection may represent real progression in the fight against HIV and AIDS. The question for many people though is whether or not this can be sustained?

Terminal care

Providing support to patients who wish to die at home

Terminal care is the very essence of general practice and once again support can only occur where there is familiarity with the individual, his or her informal 'family' network and their surroundings. It has been known for a long time that this is often an area where choice is very limited, and where patients are often kept in hospital unnecessarily and home care cannot (or will not) be arranged.

Where there is commitment from the patient's general practitioner, the hospital services and the wider primary care team, terminal care at home *is* possible. The obvious advantages to care at home are that the surroundings are familiar, care is invariably personal and there is a feeling of control by the patient in what is such a critical stage of their life.

The hospital service is also still very important because it provides support, so that should a crisis arise, the relevant in-patient services can be accessed. Sometimes, however, due to various factors, hospitals do not always fully appreciate the extent to which people with serious ailments can be supported and monitored in the community. Where the patient has developed an intercurrent problem, for example a chest infection that warrants aggressive therapy, an emergency admission to the hospital can be arranged.

A key service which is more common in urban areas is the hospice or HIV/AIDS palliative care team (Smits et al. 1990). Although hospices provide specialist palliative care service (in-patient and sometimes as day care), they vary in their extent in responding to people with HIV and AIDS. Where the service is based in a generic, non-specialist hospice, it used to be the case that referrals could only be accepted if the patient with HIV/AIDS had Kaposi's sarcoma or some other tumour.

In some larger cities like London, special hospices have been established, and some of them high profile, in order to try and meet the needs of people with HIV infection. These hospice units provide a mixture of residential care, home-based social support and day care. Perhaps the most prominent of these are London Lighthouse, based in West London, and the Mildmay Mission hospital in East London (see p. 194). Throughout the country there are four specialist HIV/AIDS residential care units, the other two being in Brighton and Edinburgh.

As stated in Chapter 4 the individual facets of terminal care are:

• Symptom control
• Avoidance of inappropriate therapy
• Support
• Multidisciplinary approach
• Continuity of care
• Communication.

Symptom control

It is difficult to list the vast range of symptoms that an individual with advanced HIV infection and AIDS may suffer. However, a number of key 'symptom groups' will be mentioned. What is important here are the underlying principles which allow for effective terminal care for individual patients.

Pain

Pain is common, though several authors have identified that there is great variation in how common it really is (Larue et al. 1997, Haughton 1997, Sims and Moss 1991). Although this is significant it probably represents the simple fact that, sometimes pain is a difficult notion to define and even more difficult to measure (after all, in the majority of cases there are few visible markers to indicate pain).

The key to pain management is, like for all other symptoms, to find out why the pain is occurring, for example, abdominal pain in a person already taking strong analgesics (painkillers) may be due to the adverse effects of the painkillers. Thus to increase the dosage may worsen and not improve the pain.

It is important to explore the pain in detail: where is it, how long has it been there, what type of pain is it? These questions ought to help the health professional localise the pain to a particular region. Often finding out what type of pain it is (is it burning, stinging, aching?) may help to define the cause of the pain, and ultimately what to do about it. In addition, certain types of analgesics are more effective in dealing with particular types of pain. This attention to detail is designed to tailor the treatment to the particular patient and although it seems a long process, it pays dividends.

The treatment of pain ought to be planned along a step-wise or graded approach. Sometimes to help with this, an analgesic chart is used where the individual affected is invited to judge how bad the pain is; thus with a range of 1–10, a score of 1 indicates the pain is present but is mild, whereas a score of 10 indicates that the pain is almost unbearable. This is useful in order to monitor how effective is the pain relief and to monitor the progress of the patient. Clearly such an instrument is not suitable for everyone.

Although known to those who work with patients with AIDS, other health care workers increasingly recognise that pain is a highly significant feature

Table 10.1   Most common painkillers used in a step-wise fashion

Severity of pain	Type of analgesia	Side-effects
Severe	Opiate-type analgesia	Nausea, sickness, constipation
Mild-Moderate	Coproxamol*, Co-codamol, Ibuprofen (Nurofen)	Ibuprofen (Nurofen) can also irritate the stomach
Mild	Simple analgesia: Asprin or paracetamol	Aspirin may irritate the stomach

*: commonly interacts with the protease-inhibitor, Retonavir (see Chapter 8)

of advancing disease. It is therefore mandatory to try and control this whenever possible in order to preserve quality of life and well-being. As already mentioned, the presence of pain in patients with advanced HIV infection including AIDS is variable (Larue et al. 1997, Haughton 1997, Sims and Moss 1991).

In a more recent French study (Larue et al. 1997), pain was a feature in over 60 per cent of patients with HIV infection. Pain was more common for in-patients and was substantially under-recognised and thus, under-treated. This comprehensive study was conducted at various centres throughout France and involved over 300 patients with HIV or AIDS. Although nearly four out of five patients in the study group were male, it points to important findings concerning the advanced stages of HIV infection and AIDS.

Box 10.1   Key points about pain symptoms (Larue 1997)

- Pain is common and debilitating in patients with HIV/AIDS
- Pain decreases the quality of the patient's life
- Pain is seriously under-treated, *because*
- Its severity is underestimated and
- The more severe the pain, the more it is under-estimated
- There is reluctance to prescribe the strongest analgesia.

It is no accident that in the list of fundamental aspects of palliative care, symptom control is the first. It is also clear that to spend the last days or weeks in pain is both unnecessary and unacceptable, especially when this impacts on quality of life in such a big way. Significantly it is often the pain's impact on others, such as carers or partners, which is most important.

One of the most important models of pain is the bio-pyscho-social model which describes pain as having a physical component as well as an emotional component. This is not difficult to envisage since pain sustained in a stressful situation, for example, a football match, will only really come to light after the match has finished when the pain is very much worse and sometimes unbearable! Thus, if a person is tired, weak, or just unwell, any pain – whatever the cause – will appear greater and perhaps more difficult to treat. Attention to these other factors is as important as merely increasing the dose of the analgesics for the patient.

Pain in the majority of instances can be controlled though, from what has been said earlier, a number of factors may need to be taken into account.

Table 10.2   A summary of the different types of pain described in patients with AIDS (Larue et al. 1977)

Type of pain	Numbers (percentage of patients)
Gastro-intestinal/mouth	26 (33%)
Muscular	25 (32%)
Joint/bone	16 (20%)
Central nervous system (CNS)	15 (19%)
Peripheral neuropathy (usually feet or arms)	10 (13%)

One important factor worthy of mention is remaining occupied; in other words being occupied by an activity is better than being preoccupied by the pain. While this can easily be misinterpreted as distracting the person from pain, this can be a genuinely effective strategy.

Many types of pain can be controlled with an escalating range of analgesia, depending on the severity, type and the cause of the pain. Regarding the sometimes sensitive question of 'how much medication does a person in pain need?', it is very difficult not to be prescriptive here, except to say that many patients will benefit from appropriate doses of moderate (see Table 10.1) or strong analgesics (morphine) so long as it is taken regularly throughout the day as recommended. What is appropriate can only be determined by the patient feeling the pain, and there is a saying in palliative care: 'the patient needs as much as the patient needs'. Different people will have different pain thresholds. In addition, pain can change and therefore it is necessary to monitor and reassess patients, especially if they are taking opiate-type analgesics such as morphine.

Patients become used to (also known as developing a tolerance to) some analgesics, especially opiates, thus increasing doses are usually needed over long periods of time. This factor is particularly important for people who use opiates (including injectables) since they will invariably need higher doses and there may be some reluctance to prescribe because of the fear of abuse. This is a difficult problem to resolve and can only be done with clinicians who have experience of these particular problems or with the help of expert advice.

Finally, medications can be prescribed which act as 'adjuncts' to actual analgesic medication, thus relieving some if not all aspects of the pain. An example here is the use of aspirin for joint/bone pain which can be used in conjunction with opiates (that is, morphine) with good effect. Anti-depressants have a useful role to play in HIV and AIDS; however, their use in advanced HIV disease, particularly terminal care, is debatable. What is known is that patients entering the final phase of the condition will often – not surprisingly and quite appropriately – be depressed. This may be regarded as part of the normal acceptance process associated with 'death and dying'. While this period is undoubtedly sad and full of sorrow, for some patients it may be a relief or they may experience a feeling of impending 'release'. This is why it is fundamental that no assumptions are made especially at such critical times for the patient. It is often helpful for the patient to be able to talk about and to articulate fears, concerns and anxieties at this time. Sometimes it is genuinely difficult to be able to distinguish sadness from depression and here trying to provide optimal care should take this uncertainty into account. A useful pointer here is the familiarity of the clinician with the patient. Often it is this knowledge, gained through experience and 'continuity of care' that helps to distinguish between what may be a passing phase of sadness with that of a more serious depressive episode.

Furthermore, the issues for people who are seen to be marginal to society, for example, gay men or injecting drug-users, may be compounded by extra feelings of anger, guilt or rage because of their overall non-acceptance. Often this marginality has been life-long and it is only now, in the last few weeks or even days, that friends and family have become aware of their loved one being gay, or an injecting drug-user.

In such painful circumstances, whether a course of anti-depressants may alleviate these feelings is unknown, though intuitively it appears highly unlikely. Many clinicians use anti-depressants in a host of settings, including the community, the hospital and the hospice; however, their overall effectiveness in this type of circumstance remains unknown.

Two important points about anti-depressants need highlighting. First, no anti-depressant will work right away – they take approximately two weeks before the earliest effect, because they need to cross the blood–brain barrier, though some of the newer formulations (for example, Prozac) may act more quickly. Furthermore, anti-depressants are often used for two indications at the same time. Thus a patient may be suffering with longstanding neuro-pathic pains and is, not surprisingly, depressed. A course of anti-depressants (ie amitryptiline) may benefit on these two counts simultaneously. Second, most clinicians advocate a long course, perhaps a few months for proper efficacy. Thus a person entering the very last stages of the condition will not benefit from medication and is more likely to suffer with adverse effects, for example a dry mouth, constipation, blurred vision or headaches. It makes sense therefore to withhold this on the basis that it will probably do more harm than good. The final arbiter in these difficult situations should clearly be the individual patient.

Many would argue that 'giving something is better than giving nothing'; however, this is poor clinical medicine. In the last stages of any condition, and HIV/AIDS is no different, the greatest requirements for the patient are often time, space for reflection and the reassurance that someone is at hand. The other person may be called upon to do very little, except perhaps the most important function, to be there. There is no end to the mystery and fear which surrounds death, a process which is becoming more and more remote as time goes on, not only from the perspective of the individual as life expectation increases but also from a social perspective as death increasingly takes place in an institutional setting, such as a hospital or hospice.

Use of analgesics (painkillers)   A couple of points need to be made about the commonest analgesics. It is sensible to start off with the simple analgesics, for example aspirin or paracetamol. Both are equally effective, although aspirin is particularly good for muscular or deep bone pains. Many patients feel that this type of analgesia will not be effective partly because it can be obtained over-the-counter from any chemist or supermarket.

These common painkillers, if taken in the right doses, can be remarkably efficient in reducing pain. In addition both of these analgesics can reduce fevers and chills very rapidly. The big problem with aspirin is that many patients have difficulty in tolerating large doses because it irritates the stomach, thus causing discomfort, heartburn or indigestion or even a combination of all three. Often this can be minimised if the aspirin is taken with or after food. If it still cannot be tolerated, paracetamol is worth a trial, since this is much less of an irritant to the stomach.

Morphine is the strongest analgesic known and has a particular place in terminal conditions generally. Many types of preparations are available, for example ordinary oral preparations, suppositories, long-acting formulations and long-acting skin patches. The actual choice for the person is one of preference, however, it is fair to say that one of the best, traditional ways of taking morphine is every four hours by mouth. The advantage of this is that regular amounts – which have been titrated beforehand – are used to maintain constant levels of analgesia in the blood, thus reducing both the pain and the fear of pain.

Critically, while it is easy to assume that delivery of morphine by injection, for example intramuscularly or intravenously, may be more effective, there is little to support this view. Thus the oral form is by far the most commonly prescribed form of analgesia for patients who need palliative care. However, where pain control is difficult or is worsening, especially if it appears to be 'out of control', intramuscular (im) injections are a way of regaining that control quickly and effectively. In such circumstances this is entirely appropriate. It should be possible therefore to restore the morphine to the oral formulation once the pain is under control, usually with higher doses. This interlude may also be appropriate if the patient is suffering with nausea and vomiting and there is a danger that further doses of oral morphine may exacerbate this.

Where morphine is used, it is important to acknowledge that nausea, vomiting and constipation are side-effects which can be severe and can actually cause more suffering. Many clinicians give anti-sickness medication with the morphine and, importantly, a laxative to counter constipation which, again, can be severe. Many clinicians would agree that a regular anti-sickness medication should be used routinely (certainly for the first few days) *and* a regular laxative be given in order to prevent morphine-induced constipation. It is wise to anticipate these effects in order to prevent the problems arising in the first place.

Weight loss

Weight loss is another common feature which occurs at any time during the course of HIV infection, in other words in early or late stages of the condition. As with pain, it is always necessary to try and identify why this is happening, and seeking the advice of the clinician is important. The causes of weight loss are multiple and range from the simple, lack of appetite due to an associated depressive illness to infection-associated diarrhoea and vomiting (Summerbell 1994). Simple problems, for example mouth ulcers or persistent oral thrush, can severely reduce a patient's intake of food remarkably quickly. Of course, these are treatable in the majority of cases.

Perhaps the most important intervention, taking the cause into account, is to seek the advice of a specialist dietician who could provide input (see Chapter 7).

Disfigurement

Disfigurement can be a feature of HIV and AIDS for some of the reasons that have already been mentioned. A person affected by advanced HIV infection and suffering with Kaposi's sarcoma (KS) can be doubly affected, since these are perceived to be the 'tell-tale' lesions and are often, cruelly, in prominent places such as the face, forehead or nose. Although a number of these problems can be ameliorated, unfortunately there is no cure (see Chapter 3 for the range of available treatment options). Thus, for the person affected, this disfigurement is both cruel and tragic and may well represent a rapid transition from living with HIV/AIDS to dying from it.

It is difficult to know what is best at this point in time. Often the patient will be in a better position to decide what the options are at this point, usually with advice from partner, friends or family. It should be clear that the disfigurement is much more than a simple 'bodily change', but more of a symbolic threat to the 'real' self and it is not at all surprising that patients like this suffer profound depression, often are socially withdrawn and may express suicidal thoughts (see Chapter 5).

Cough

Coughing may be a problem in the pre-terminal stages; however, it ought to figure less during the actual terminal stages of the disease. One of the reasons for this may be that the stronger analgesics – such as morphine – have anti-cough (called antitussive) actions. One of the more common problems, especially in the last few hours, and sometimes days, is a nasty 'rattle' of the chest which may be a harbinger of the death itself. While sometimes distressing for the patient it is always distressing for relatives and loved ones. It can be diminished rapidly with hyoscine, a medication designed to reduce the secretions ordinarily produced by the respiratory system. If very bad or immediate relief is required, an injection of hyoscine can produce relief within minutes.

Agitation and terminal restlessness

These are the names given to the general restlessness that sometimes accompanies the final stages of the terminal illness. The points made earlier about trying to identify the reason are still valid – is the patient in pain? are they constipated? or just very frightened? Usually at such a late stage the patient will be 'unconscious', however, the agitation can still be very alarming for all concerned. The treatment of the agitation is relatively easy although a number of therapeutic options are available. For example, increasing the dose of opiates may well be appropriate, since this is naturally sedating. The addition of diazepam (Valium) in order to increase sedation may be warranted. Another type of medication, exemplified by drugs such as chlorpromazine or haloperidol, also induce sedation when given orally, though injection (sub-cutaneous, via the skin) is a possibility. One feature of this stage may be the presence of 'Cheyne-Stokes' breathing which arises when the level of consciousness drops further. It is characterised by a cyclical variation in breathing ranging from periods of quite rapid breathing (hyperpnoea) to long periods without a breath (apnoea). This breathing can last for many hours and only really occurs in the period immediately preceding death.

Nevertheless, because patients with AIDS are relatively young, this latter phase may last many hours if not days, in contrast to the elderly where there is not so much reserve and is therefore much shorter.

Decreasing mobility

The causes of decreasing mobility are many and trying to determine the main reason is difficult but can prove to be useful. The obvious ones include sensory impairment, for example reduced vision, or other neurological problems. The latter group can be sub-divided into causes related to motor nerve dysfunction, spinal cord disorders and finally, central control problems such as ataxia (inability to walk in a straight line). This latter group are called central nervous system problems. Motor nerves are the nerves which supply the muscles of the body and which are under conscious control.

Thus a 'motor nerve lesion' usually affects limb function such as the arms or legs. It is sometimes difficult to discern whether it is HIV infection or a manifestation of AIDS, which is the causal factor. Moreover, such symptoms such as a tingling in the feet or hands (peripheral neuropathy) may be also due to an adverse effect of one of the medications designed to counteract the underlying HIV/AIDS.

Certainly, some of the newer anti-HIV medications can cause a neurological sensory neuropathy, that is, a sensation of pins and needles in arms and legs which can be debilitating. It is always prudent to seek advice about this, since some medications may need to be decreased or should be stopped before the neuropathy becomes worse and permanent. It is important to note that in the advanced stages of the condition, that a combination of these factors may all contribute to the decreasing mobility of the affected patient. Where this is the case, the full range of the multidisciplinary team becomes involved, bringing with them their special expertise and knowledge in the various areas.

Quality of life

At such a juncture in a patient's illness it is quality of life that is the key factor. How a patient judges their life to have sufficient quality is very much a personal, individualised and sometimes unpredictable affair. Health care professionals need to know and acknowledge this, perhaps explicitly with the patient. If the subject is approached professionally and sensitively, the person can adjust relatively smoothly to an increasingly advanced stage of HIV infection. It should be the case that all such health professionals can deal with advanced-stage disease properly and professionally. Where this is not the case it is incumbent upon those responsible (ultimately the health care workers themselves) to ensure training and education is provided. Why is this?

Very simply the majority of patients who are suffering such conditions know that this is so. Whether they choose to articulate it is another matter. However one of the reasons why patients choose not to articulate their fears about impending death is that they fear their health worker will not be able to cope with these frank discussions. These intimate conversations, talking openly about patient's worst fears, the effects it will have on others, hopes for the children and death itself, are some of the most difficult and yet paradoxically the most satisfying (for the health professionals).

Case history

A 42-year old man, AB, with HIV and AIDS lives with his long-standing partner in a flat in South-east London. He has been diagnosed with HIV infection seven years ago and an AIDS diagnosis was made following confirmation of Kaposi's sarcoma in his lungs three years ago. Over the past year or so, he has generally deteriorated in that he was diagnosed with pneumocystis carinii pneumonia (PCP) and had a number of other chest infections. He has been in and out of hospital, in this case a major London teaching hospital, in the past twelve months.

He has deteriorated in a number of ways, for example, he has continued to lose weight, is breathless even while almost at rest and he feels tired and listless the majority of the time. He knows, though rarely admits it to himself or others, that he is entering the advanced stages of AIDS. One of his most distressing symptoms is haemoptysis, or 'coughing up' blood which is characteristic of Kaposi's sarcoma (KS) in the lung. He is cared for at home by his partner, who works in the City and thus the last few weeks have been a strain, both on AB as well as his partner.

There are support services, for example district nurses visit, though this is largely governed by AB. AB continues to visit the hospital clinic for courses of intravenous chemotherapy injections two or three times each week for Kaposi's sarcoma.

Emotionally, AB does not feel ready to give up the struggle, hoping for a remission in his symptoms. Thus up until recently he was on Zidovudine (AZT), Didanosine (ddI) and a newer type of medication, called a protease inhibitor (Retonavir).

It is the hospital clinicians who are most involved with AB, and he has seen a succession of counsellors during his treatments, mostly at his out-patient attendances. AB's general practitioner (GP) has been kept informed of the various changes to his medications, as well as his overall progress. Indeed, it was the GP, who, after a frank discussion with AB, admitted him to hospital during his last episode. At this time, AB's breathing was distressingly worse and he had suffered another heavy bout of haemoptysis, which frightened him even more.

Following his last admission to hospital, AB was unusually keen to anticipate what would happen in the near future, in effect to plan his own death. He had several discussions with his partner and his mother, who up until now had played a significant though 'backroom' role in his overall care. He finally decided that there was little point in continuing to pursue the punishing systemic chemotherapy, which he confessed made his tiredness even worse. However, he did not give up the Zidovudine, Didanosine or the Retonavir.

Although he had been on slow-release morphine (called MST or Morphine Sustained Release), he was switched to oral morphine every four hours so that an overall dosage could be properly calculated.

AB's distress, his breathing problems and the pain he suffered from previous genital KS, made morphine the most appropriate of medications to be used. As a precaution he was also given a laxative in order to prevent constipation secondary to the morphine.

After four days, in which his breathing improved substantially, albeit temporarily, he died peacefully, surrounded by his partner, his mother and close friends. During the last 24 hours, he had a sub-cutaneous morphine pump which ensured that he received the same pain relief even though he could not swallow.

Avoidance of inappropriate therapy

It is a challenge for health professionals, and more importantly for the person affected, to know what is appropriate therapy and thus, what is inappropriate. Logically this can be extended to any intervention; what is appropriate may well appear inappropriate the following day. Sometimes it is impossible to distinguish between the two.

The reason this is mentioned in this section is that many of us on the health professional side of the relationship have seen and witnessed interventions carried out on patients which, no matter how viewed, cannot be in the patient's best interests. This is why this ethical minefield is a particularly sensitive one to cross.

In the end who is responsible for making such important decisions? Of course, and almost without saying, it should be the patient with HIV or AIDS who is informed and consents to treatment or not as the case may be. In the case history above, AB had decided for himself that, while a trial of anti-retroviral therapies was worthwhile, for him it was not worth pushing this – and punishing himself – endlessly.

Of course the interests of the family or partner, the agenda of the various doctors and the psycho-emotional state of the person affected will influence the patient in significant ways. In many ways AB made this decision easy for all: he had weighed up the benefits and the problems, which to a large extent was based on experience, and had decided to stop all therapy including the anti-retroviral medications.

At the end of this chapter there is a full description of living wills and advanced directives which can help to facilitate key decisions about what is and is not appropriate for patients with HIV infection.

Support

Irrespective of 'stage of illness' the role of the visiting health professional is to try to help and support the person affected by HIV and AIDS. Often it is not just the patient who requires help, but also individual family members, the partner or close friends. This facet of care is perhaps more visible if the patient is being cared for at home, although not always. One area which is often overlooked, especially at such emotionally charged times, is the spiritual care of the person and/or family members.

Because HIV and AIDS are still highly stigmatised conditions, general support often requires much forethought. In the larger cities it tends to be less of a problem, especially if contacts are made with recognised voluntary organisations such as the Terence Higgins Trust. Interestingly, in the case of AB, although he knew about the many agencies in the London area, he preferred to cope without this form of support. He was heavily reliant on his partner and latterly on the many health care workers who came to his aid.

The continuing diversification of people being affected by HIV and AIDS, for example ethnic minority groups and women, means that support groups and networks may not be as well-developed as in the more traditional groups such as gay men. Sustained support remains a major need for those affected by this condition.

Multidisciplinary approach

It has already been stated that to provide good, effective, sensitive care to people approaching the end of their lives with HIV and AIDS requires the full range of the primary care team's help (see Chapter 4). Not only the doctor can provide a range of medical services, the clinician can call upon the services of palliative care specialists, district nurses and MacMillan nurses in order to ensure care is comprehensive.

In the case of AB, following several of his earlier discharges from hospital, an occupational therapist accompanied him home to ensure that he could carry out basic activities of daily living. Although he did not need to have many physical adaptations to the flat, AB was advised about a number of aspects in the flat (Cusack 1994). It needs to be stated, however, that adaptations can be expensive and usually, depending on the financial position in the locality, there may be a waiting list for such arrangements.

The role of a physiotherapist is potentially wide, though changing. Initially, within the HIV/AIDS context, their role was 'systems'-based, for example looking after patients requiring prophylaxis against pneumocystis carinii pneumonia. This was common some years ago when the prophylaxis of PCP was with pentamidine, a medication which was delivered through special inhalers called nebulisers. By contrast the physiotherapist's role has become more holistic; thus they are more active in rehabilitation, pain management, minimising disability and facilitating exercise schemes (McClure 1994).

The role of voluntary organisations is immensely important. Depending on the available resources, they can provide a whole series of services and facilities to aid the person affected in their own home. In larger cities such as London or Edinburgh, there are 'drop-in' centres which have on-site crèche facilities, a cafe providing subsidised meals as well as other more formal services. One very large London facility prides itself on a locally-based group of specially trained volunteers who provide ongoing support of a practical nature to people and families with HIV infection or AIDS. The aim of this service is to complement other statutory services in order to ensure that quality of life is maintained for as long as possible. This practical help may range from cleaning and clearing up, to preparing food or perhaps helping with personal cleaning and hygiene. These community volunteers are called 'helpers', support staff, or 'buddies', the latter term reflecting that it is also the emotional help which is valued as much as the practical.

For people who require ongoing help, support in the form of a generic social worker is invaluable. Their professional role is a cocktail of health and social, welfare rights, counsellor and personal friend and no less valued for it (Bairstow 1994). Often their role is to organise a package of care which is specifically tailored to a particular patient. Although their roles are forever changing, they are often in the invidious position whereby too little or too much intervention attracts criticism way beyond what is reasonable. They are often called upon to perform in the most trying of circumstances with the most challenging of patients in an environment where resources are inevitably constrained.

Continuity of care

From the patient's point of view, 'continuity of care' is seen to be a vital component of care and if a series of impersonal, ever-changing number of health workers try to provide support, they are likely to fail for obvious reasons. One of the reasons that health care works in general practice is that the relationship between patient and primary care team is close, sustained and familiar.

From the health professional point of view, continuity is genuinely difficult to provide, due to various factors such as working shifts, changing surgery times and the non-complementary style of care workers.

The other point to make here is that people have extremely variable perceptions of what constitutes continuity of care. For example, many patients who attend hospital departments complain about 'never seeing the same doctor twice', but others say exactly the same of their GP surgery – especially if the latter is large. Much of this is, ultimately, about personal circumstance and individual expectations. Many patients, especially in the advanced stages of disease will be familiar with their own local general practitioner and primary care team, including district nurse and perhaps liaison support nurse (palliative or specialist). The main role of hospital-based palliative care home support teams is to bridge the inevitable gap which exists between the hospital and home where such intensive support can never emulate that in the hospital. One particular strength of home support teams is that, in an ideal world, they can almost start planning discharge arrangements as soon as the patient is admitted. The team can be likened to 'a stepping stone' from the more intensive hospital-based care to more informal, less rigid home care.

Unfortunately, with the changes in 24-hour cover in general practice, out-of-hours care (after 7 p.m. and through the night until the following morning, and weekends) can be more problematic at times. Having stated this it is important to realise that teams such as this discuss how best to cope with such out-of-hours needs, and, for example, what to do in an emergency should this occur at the weekend.

Communication

Once again the central key to effective care apart from planning, organisation and attention to detail is communication between all members of the team. How this is done is extremely variable and has more to do with local knowledge and traditions.

The usual form of communication about patients is through the hospital or clinic letter, though how quickly (or slowly) this arrives in the community is determined by a host of factors. Where there is obvious urgency, clinicians can communicate by telephone, although this is generally under-used by all. The advent of modern forms of information technology is beginning to impact on services. A trial of instant communication using faxes and mobile phones in West London was successful though whether this can be sustained in all parts of the country is open to debate (Smith et al. 1996).

Interestingly, this last study proved that the more modern forms of communication can and arguably ought to be used to a greater extent. Thus, the clinicians routinely faxed letters of discharge on the same day that patients left the ward to return home. In addition, the hospital consultants were available to the general practitioners on a 24-hour basis through a special mobile phone number which was printed on each discharge summary. The evaluation of this research was very positive, with greater continuity of care clearly being delivered to patients with HIV infection and AIDS.

At this point it is necessary to state that communication with and for the person affected by HIV or AIDS is an absolute must. The days of medical paternalism when doctors or health professionals made decisions for the patient (often without them even knowing about it!) – are now fast receding. It is now reasonable to expect that a decision regarding a person's care ought to be made with the person at the heart of that process. This is the true meaning of informed consent: consent to an intervention which is based upon a true understanding of the benefits and problems associated with a particular course of action. As part of this process, the health professional (including hospital doctor or general practitioner) ought to be able to provide alternatives and perhaps options, although it is important to remember that a GP's knowledge is *general*, thus not of a specialist kind. Of course, where necessary, the specialist and the generalist will communicate about difficult problems, in a manner in common with many other conditions.

Sometimes communication between health professionals is difficult because there is often not one single forum where all groups meet (doctors, nurses, therapists). In order to counteract this, a booklet can be left with the patient – which has the advantage that the care worker records the outcome of their latest consultation – so that other visitors to the home can leave a record of their visit. This model works well in some circumstances.

Living wills and advanced directives

Perhaps not surprisingly, there is growing interest in living wills and advanced directives (Schlyter 1992); these are instruments whereby patients with serious diseases – irrespective of type – can inform medical and nursing staff how they wish to be treated if they were to become so seriously ill that they were not in a position to make a decision. In the context of HIV/AIDS, an example would be if a patient was admitted to an intensive care unit having suddenly collapsed on account of an AIDS-related pneumonia.

A living will is usually a written statement setting out the patient's wishes regarding life-sustaining treatment. It can also provide more general advice such as which types of treatment will be accepted and also which types will be rejected in certain circumstances. It is a condition of the statement that the person 'is of sound mind' when it was signed. In addition it will only be consulted in the event that the person cannot communicate his or her wishes. Actual copies of such a document can be obtained from the Terence Higgins Trust (see 'Useful Addresses' at the end of this volume).

Another way of providing this information is to appoint someone, either a family member, partner or good friend who would act as a *proxy*, in such dire circumstances. They are then acting as an *enduring power of attorney* for health care. It is interesting to note that there is no formal legislation in the United Kingdom which allows the appointment of a power of attorney for health care, though there is one for property.

Clearly, living wills are potentially useful, both in terms of maximising communication between patient and doctor and allowing discussions about sensitive and difficult subjects to be more explicit. Of course the majority of health care professionals would, if a living will was present, take this into account (indeed they would probably be relieved to know that the issues had been discussed).

A High Court ruling concluded that advance directives by patients about future interventions are legally binding (Dyer 1993). Another advantage for the patient is that they decide for themselves the extent to which complications should or should not be treated, in a way which maximises control over the condition. It is often this lack of control which makes conditions like HIV and AIDS so frightening.

One of the concerns for doctors, and nurses to some extent, is that the patient may have changed their minds in these new circumstances. Moreover, especially where a number of close friends, including the patient's partner, may be involved, sorting out disagreements may be more troublesome than first envisaged. However, in one of the most comprehensive studies carried out in the UK, it was felt that a living will would be beneficial in four different ways:

1 It would facilitate more explicit discussions about sensitive issues such as life-sustaining interventions, including treatments. This is much

easier if a set pro forma is used which then informs the health professional that the issue has been explored prior to seeing the doctor or nurse.

2   It is clear that one of the main advantages of such an instrument is that it allows the patient much more control over their destiny than would be possible without a directive. This control is appreciated by such groups as the Terence Higgins Trust who firmly believe that the time is ripe for living wills and advanced directives to play a major role in the care of people with HIV and AIDS.

3   Such a living directive may also clarify who are the important 'significant others' in attempting to determine what is the best overall course of action for a patient.

4   Lastly, such an instrument would perhaps reduce the stress and pressure from those closest to the patient, especially where such life-determining decisions needed to be made. Once again, knowing that the patient had carefully considered, taken advice and signed the relevant documents while competent, indicates that his or her wishes were the main motivating factor from the start of the process (Schlyter 1992).

Summary

In this chapter the principles of providing good, effective palliative care are described and explored. For those working in primary care, much pride can be taken in the fact that care can be accessible, flexible, patient-centred and locally based. For the patient with HIV infection or AIDS, the benefits of this local service working alongside the specialist care centres can pay dividends in many different ways.

In the special case of a person suffering with advancing HIV disease it is palliative care which is the most critical aspect of the ongoing care. There is the imperative to ensure that the patient can be maintained in comfort and in familiar surroundings for as long as the disease process allows.

One facet of this care, that is pain control, is duly emphasised, because it is still under-recognised and under-treated. Most importantly, in all of these processes, it is the patient's choice and control which ultimately control – or should at any rate – how this care is delivered.

Doctors, nurses and the whole health care team ought to be orchestrated by the complex needs of the patient. Where, due to a variety of circumstances, the patient cannot do this, or needs to do this accompanied, the process may be slower but no less intense for all concerned. Where the patient cannot decide due to serious or severe disease, pre-planning with the establishment of an advanced directive or a living will may identify who is the real advocate for the patient. This person can play a highly significant role in the major decisions which often need to be made in the last few hours or days of life.

References

Bairstow, S. (1994) 'The social worker's role in HIV' in Cusack, L. and Singh, S. (eds), *HIV and AIDS Care – practical approaches*, London: Chapman and Hall.

Cusack, L. (1994) 'The role of the Occupational Therapist' in Cusack, L. and Singh, S. (eds) *HIV and AIDS Care – practical approaches*, London: Chapman and Hall.

Dyer, C. (1993) 'High court says advance directives are binding', *British Medical Journal*, 307: 1023–4.

Haughton, N. (1997) 'Management of HIV/AIDS in general practice', London: BMA Foundation for AIDS.

King, M. (1993) *AIDS, HIV and Mental Health*, Cambridge: Cambridge University Press.

Larue, F., Fontaine, A. and Colleau, S. (1997) 'Underestimation and undertreatment of pain in HIV disease: multicentre study', *British Medical Journal*, 314: 23–8.

Mansfield, S. and Singh, S. (1990) 'The management of HIV/AIDS in primary care', London: BMA Foundation for AIDS.

McClure, J. (1994) 'The role of the physiotherapist', in Cusack, L. and Singh, S. (eds) *HIV and AIDS Care – practical approaches*, London: Chapman and Hall.

OHE (Office of Health Economics) (1991) 'Dying with dignity', No. 97 in a series of reports about health problems, London: OHE.

Schlyter, C. (1992) *Advance directives & AIDS: an empirical study of the interest in living wills and proxy decision making in the context of HIV/AIDS care*, London: Centre of Medical Law and Ethics.

Sims, R. and Moss, V. (1991) *Terminal care for people with AIDS*, London: Edward Arnold Publishers.

Smith, S., Robinson, J., Hollyer et al. (1996) 'Combining specialist and primary health care teams for HIV positive patients: retrospective and prospective studies', *British Medical Journal*, 312: 416–20.

Smits, A., Mansfield S. and Singh, S. (1990) 'Facilitating care of patients with HIV infection by hospital and primary care teams', *British Medical Journal*, 300: 241–2.

Summerbell, C. (1994) 'Nutrition in HIV disease' in Cusack, L. and Singh, S. (eds) *HIV and AIDS Care – practical approaches*, London: Chapman and Hall.

11 Death and its Related Processes

This chapter covers what to do after death, irrespective of where this occurs, and includes an explanation of the necessary administrative tasks. The section also deals with death at home and some of the questions people and carers frequently ask of health care workers.

The chapter will then go on to explore how the grieving process and bereavement affects loved ones or carers before examining how this process can deviate to become 'abnormal' and require further expert help. Finally, a short analysis of how death is viewed, particularly in Western-type societies will be described and how this relates to those with HIV infection and AIDS.

What to do when someone dies at home

When the patient dies at home, this is often the most difficult period for the carer (or carers) who have been so closely involved with looking after the person who has just died. What is there to be done? The very first task is to confirm that death has occurred and this should be carried out by a doctor. Usually this entails an examination of the chest (to check breathing and to listen to the heart) and an examination of the eyes (to check for pupil change or a 'light-reflex').

At the risk of sounding callous, the most important tasks are sorting out the death certificate and organising the funeral. The completion of the death certificate by a doctor is the main administrative task and is necessary before the body can be released for any purpose. If the certificate cannot be completed straight away, for example over a weekend the undertakers should collect the body and it will remain in a chapel of rest.

A death certificate can only be legally filled out by a practising doctor.

That doctor must be 'familiar' with the patient who has just died; in practice this means the doctor ought to have seen the patient within the last two weeks. If this is not the case, then legally the doctor cannot fill out the death certificate. The cause of death should be stated if known, and this should include HIV infection or AIDS where appropriate.

However, because HIV and AIDS are still stigmatised conditions, many clinicians are reluctant to state HIV infection or AIDS on the death certificate, even though ultimately these may have contributed to the cause of death. The simple reason for this is that a death certificate is a public document and thus available to anyone who wishes to see it. In addition the death certificate may need to be presented to a variety of agencies after death (ie employers, local authority) and hence confidentiality is broken. The distress to the relatives of the deceased may adversely affect the grieving process and is thus an important point (King 1993) (see p. 182). This is undoubtedly a controversial area; however, common courses of action are described below.

Death certification

The guidance to doctors is that cause of death ought to be stated *to the best of the doctor's knowledge and belief*. In order for this to be explored further it is necessary to know a little more about the purposes of death certification.

There are two main reasons for death certification. First, that the death is recorded and the doctor is satisfied that the deceased has not died in suspicious circumstances. Second, the certificate does form the basis – thankfully not the only basis – for epidemiological statistics about death and its various causes.

In cases where the cause of death was mysterious but not unexpected (in which case a referral to the coroner may be necessary), there is often more information which can be gleaned from a post mortem. The death certificate allows the doctor to provide further information at a later date, usually within a few days. Thus, a common occurrence in cases of HIV infection or AIDS is for the certifying doctor to state that the final illness was 'bronchopneumonia', which is usually an accurate enough description of the final illness. At the same time, the doctor states that further information will be forthcoming. A few days later the final cause of death – bronchopneumonia – will be expanded to include HIV infection and AIDS. In the meantime the death certificate issued to the relatives remains unchanged and states 'bronchopneumonia'.

A death should be reported to the coroner if, as stated above, there are suspicious circumstances of death, including possible elements of violence.

The coroner, who has a dual professional qualification – legal and medical – is a pathologist whose task it is to ascertain how and why the death occurred.

If the doctor has not seen the patient in the previous 14 days, the deceased may well become a 'coroner's case'. The onus is on the doctor to inform or liaise with the coroner if there are any queries about the death. Other reasons why the coroner ought to be informed include, for example, if the patient has died following an accident, or where death was due to neglect or self-neglect. In addition, the coroner will be alerted if there is suspicion the death was due to suicide or, in the case of a woman, if a termination of pregnancy (TOP) or abortion had recently been performed. However, there is no need to inform the coroner just because the person has died from an HIV or AIDS-related condition.

It is a good idea to contact the hospital or treatment unit so that an official notification can be made to the Public Health Laboratory Service (PHLS) about the death. Again, this last process is for statistical and epidemiological data and there is a particular emphasis on maintaining confidentiality.

Box 11.1   The death certificate

Part 1 of the certificate
- Disease stated leading to death, i.e. *bronchopneumonia*
- Sequence of diseases leading to death, i.e. *AIDS*
- Underlying cause of death may be stated on the last completed line of Part 1, i.e. *HIV infection*.

Part 2 of the certificate
- A significant condition or disease which contributed to death but is not part of any sequence leading to death, i.e. *diabetes mellitus*; this can be left blank.

If there is any doubt about the cause of death doctors will discuss this with the coroner, because it is a legal requirement. Often small queries can be sorted out over the telephone, in which case the family can be saved from further distress at a time when emotions are running high and sensitivity is required all round.

Once the death certificate has been filled out this should be delivered to the Registrar of Births and Deaths. In practice, the certificate is given to the relatives who then deliver it to the Registrar. Once this is complete the death is then officially registered. The Registrar of Births and Deaths may ask for the following documents as well as the death certificate:

- National Health Service (NHS) card
- Benefits/pension book
- Birth certificate if available.

Whoever delivers the death certificate to the Registrar will also be asked the following:

- Full name (and maiden name where appropriate) of the deceased
- Their place of birth
- Their occupation (and the occupation of widow(er))
- Their usual address
- Name and date of birth of the widow(er) where appropriate.

Some basic statistics about death

Approximately three-quarters of the 580,000 deaths in England and Wales are certified by a hospital doctor or general practitioner. The remaining quarter are certified by a coroner. In the latter case, approximately 60 per cent are voluntarily referred by a doctor, 2 per cent by a Registrar and the remaining 38 per cent from other sources, mainly the police (Office for National Statistics 1996). Some people have tried to label HIV and AIDS deaths 'unnatural' thus requiring coroner's certification; remember: *there is no need to inform the coroner merely because the person has died from an HIV or an AIDS-related condition.*

Cremation form

If the body is to be cremated, another important two-part form needs to be filled out by the doctor, usually the same doctor who signed the death certificate. In addition – and this is not special to HIV or AIDS – another doctor is called upon to sign the second part of this form. These requirements are to ensure that the final disposal of the body, in this case irretrievably, is again carried out with due care while ensuring that any suspicious circumstances are excluded. In these final arrangements, bodily appendages such as a pacemaker are removed prior to the cremation.

The 'second' doctor needs to be senior, in other words at least six years post-qualification and should not have seen the deceased when alive. This second doctor must actually *see* the body of the deceased, and have discussed with the doctor who signed the first half of the form, the circumstances of the death. Only once this has been completed will the undertakers allow the cremation to take place. Usually it is the task of the doctor who signs the death certificate to identify another physician to sign the second part of the cremation form.

In the community, and because this second doctor cannot have been involved with the care of the patient prior to death, another 'independent' doctor will be called to complete this second half of the form, for example another local GP. In a hospital setting it will be another senior doctor who has not contributed to the care of the patient prior to death.

Burial

In the case of burial there are few restrictions on the body because of HIV infection or AIDS. The Public Health Laboratory Service (PHLS) advises against embalming the body, however there should not be any other restrictions on the body just because of HIV. Obviously the virus will remain viable within the body for a certain period, perhaps up to two weeks after death; however, this does not mean it poses a high infection risk. Many 'bodies' may pose a risk of infection with a wide range of germs of all types including bacteria, viruses and fungi. It is however sensible to maintain basic safeguards, such as using gloves and aprons where handling of the body is necessary.

Guidelines to funeral directors are extremely variable and it may be wise to try and find a firm which has handled the deceased bodies of people with HIV in the past. At a time of upset and distress the last thing is to confront a funeral director who does not know how to handle such bodies, or does so only in a crass and insensitive manner. It is still not unknown for directors to attempt to 'double-bag' such bodies, which is old-fashioned and unnecessary. Further advice can be obtained from the Terence Higgins Trust (see 'Useful Addresses' at the end of this volume).

Dealing with funerals

Some people wish to organise their own funerals (McCrory 1994). Although for some this may seem strange and morbid, HIV infection and AIDS bring into sharp focus the fact that life is finite and death is the natural culmination.

As a gross generalisation, people in Western countries are not good at dealing with death and its various processes. Many people seem to deny that death occurs at all and even if it does, then it affects 'others'. Socio-historically in the West, people are less adept at dealing with death, probably because the expectation is that the majority of individuals will live out their 'three score years and ten'. It is important to remember this expectation is a relatively recent phenomena.

The information in this section is based upon a very useful leaflet entitled 'Dealing with Funerals' written by Paul McCrory and printed by Body Positive, London. A number of salient points in the leaflet are very sensible and very practical. Its main advantage is that the author explores these issues as someone with HIV infection and as someone who has attended many funerals.

The main organisational requirements can be summarised as follows:

- Simplicity works the best. The whole event can be likened to a (farewell) party and thus the venue and content needs to be fully considered, especially if time is a big factor.
- The instructions for these arrangements need to be clear and concise. They ought to be formalised and finalised as part of the will, or better still, constitute a separate document to be left with the executor of the will or with family and friends. These documents are not legally binding; however, if recorded, they are invariably 'morally binding'. Disputes ought to be resolved prior to death, and if necessary, with arbitration, in order to allow for a smooth period immediately after the death.
- Because any funeral is a powerful event, taking advice about it is prudent and wise. It may also help to prevent the disputes which were hinted at in the last paragraph. Sadly, these do happen. One of the most important considerations here is whether the ultimate cause of death – HIV or AIDS – is or ought to be common knowledge. If at all possible, it is sensible not to leave a discussion about this to the last moment, since those closest to the dying person may feel extraordinarily traumatised if this revelation is made at the end of their life.
- Any good, competent undertaker ought to be able to provide guidance on this subject. Some firms, especially in the larger cities, are becoming expert in organising funerals for young people who have died of AIDS-related disorders.
- The financial cost of a funeral should never be underestimated. Although this appears to be an insensitive time to discuss this aspect, it is better to acknowledge this early on. While a small state subsidy is allowed if the deceased was on Income Support in the UK, the cost for the funeral is recuperated from 'the estate'.
- Probably the most significant event in the overall proceedings will be determined by whether the body is buried or cremated. Burial charges are slightly higher, and graves invariably require maintenance. Cremation charges arise from the time allocated at the crematorium

and for the process of incineration. In this last case, some people request that the ashes be transported to or scattered in a particular location. Certain religious beliefs request that the ashes or the corpse be transported to specific locations (see the case history of TD, p. 181).

● In many cases people specifically request that the funeral be not so much a final good-bye but rather a celebration of a life, albeit one that has been unfulfilled. This will result in quite different proceedings with the ambience, the atmosphere and the overall content being quite dissimilar to an ordinary funeral. Thus, details such as the final venue (church, crematorium, house), and the type of service (religious or not, final farewell, celebration) will help decide how long the oration ought to be. Clearly the 'minister', of whatever denomination, ought to be helpful regarding this aspect of his or her work and may even organise the whole event, if this is what is requested. In a non-religious event, the lead person can be chosen by the deceased and may be a family member or even the executor of the will.

For those determined to finish positively, if that is possible in these circumstances, a wake may be appropriate, but will need organising. Once again the venue ought to be considered as well as geographic location and whether refreshments (including alcohol) will be available or not.

The social functions of such events should not be underestimated and many argue – especially anthropologists – that it is the social cohesion that is manifest at such times which is all powerful.

● Some people are determined that no flowers are sent, but rather that donations are given to worthwhile causes such as HIV/AIDS charities, other notable causes or a church of whatever denomination.

Post mortem

One of the most common reactions to a request or even an impending request for a post-mortem is 'what good can it possibly do at this stage?'

On the more positive side, some patients want the opportunity to ensure that the clinicians continue to learn about the natural history and pathology of HIV/AIDS, and specifically request a post mortem. Where there is an absolute commitment to this and the individual has had the foresight to plan it, this request may be formalised and written into the living will (see Chapter 10).

Especially where the final process is unknown, or there is something clinically unusual about the final illness, the hospital doctors usually request a post mortem. The main advantage for the clinicians is that they have the opportunity to explore and examine in detail the pathological processes which resulted in death. This may also be important for family members, especially if the clinicians were not able to clarify certain features. Theoretically, it may be beneficial for further patients with similar illnesses in the future who present in similar ways. Some say that a post mortem is always helpful since AIDS is a relatively new set of conditions and the full range of associated pathologies have yet to be fully ascertained. Post mortems do have their disadvantages, especially for the family or loved ones. For example, it may delay the funeral arrangements or the family may be so upset by the prospect of a post mortem that they cannot possibly conceive of a possible benefit. In these latter circumstances it is not surprising if families, relatives or loved ones politely refuse.

Some people believe that the appearance of the deceased will be so distorted as to make them unrecognisable if a post mortem is carried out. The mortician and pathologist are usually only too aware of such issues and every attempt will be made to ensure that incisions and scars are kept to an absolute minimum. Usually, once completed the body will look as if it has not been tampered with, except at very close inspection. If the body is fully dressed, there will be minimal exposure of the skin surfaces so that little will remain visible. If the body is lightly dressed according to cultural and religious beliefs, this may present more of a problem and therefore should be fully discussed before a final decision is made about a post mortem.

Finally, in the hospital setting, the request for a post mortem is often one of the most difficult ones for a junior doctor to make. It is always more appropriate for the request to come from a senior doctor; however, usually it is devolved to a more junior member of the team (Turner and Raphael 1997).

Where no formal instructions exists, the family or those recently bereaved ought to make this decision without undue pressure or coercion. If a post-mortem is agreed, all well and good; if the decision is no, this ought to be accepted by all concerned.

Location and death

Much of what has been stated in the sections above apply to wherever the patient has died, whether this is at home, in a hospital or in a hospice. The only difference is that it is much more unlikely that a post mortem will be requested outside of a hospital, though general practitioners have been known to request a post mortem in the community, albeit rarely. The guidelines for death certification are no different if the patient dies in a hospice. Sometimes if only a very short time is spent in the hospice before the patient dies, then it may be necessary to involve the general practitioner, especially if the latter has been seeing the patient quite regularly.

Culture and death

As can be seen from the last section the requests and requirements of those recently bereaved will be dependent on many factors, of which culture is one. Culture here means many, diverse and often interrelated notions, not merely a person's religious or ethnic background. The following case history provides a good example.

Case history

A 50-year-old Greek businessman, TD, was admitted to a residential unit in London following a number of AIDS-related opportunistic infections. He had spent the last two months on an acute HIV/AIDS ward at a central London teaching hospital. After a short period of remission, he died in the residential unit. He spent his last week, when his strength allowed, attempting to finalise a number of administrative tasks. Although the majority of his family were in Greece, he had a younger brother in the UK who was a teacher. Apparently, although this could never be verified, most of his family did not know that he was gay, and certainly did not know he was HIV-positive or that he had AIDS. The one exception to this was his younger brother.

After TD's death, his brother requested that his body be transported to Greece. This proved to be quite a challenge. Although this man was not religious in any significant way his brother explained that the body ought to be returned to his home village where he had spent much of his childhood. Thus, social and cultural factors appeared to be the main reasons for this request. The death certificate was duly filled out by the medical officer on the residential unit. The back of the certificate was also filled out allowing further information to be passed to the Registrar at a later date, which in this case was within the same week.

The major task of transporting the body to Greece was then undertaken. In essence this could not have been carried out without the help of a specialist undertaker who had done this previously. The body was prepared and then hermetically sealed within the coffin before being transported via an airliner to Greece. The main barrier to this overall procedure was the cost. However, since this was a genuine last request and TD was a fairly affluent businessman, ultimately the finances were not a big problem. The whole process was completed within a few days.

The main point behind this case history is that where possible, planning and anticipation were the keys to ensure his 'return' to Greece. In other words, it is possible that a type of protocol can be established such that a specialist undertaker is identified before the event, and not after when emotions will be running high, and usually when decisions need to be made rapidly. It is important to note that it is only with the help of such undertakers that customs clearance will be carried out smoothly. At a time like this it is inadvisable for such critical issues (or the relevant forms) to be forgotten, since it will destroy any semblance of organisation and more seriously, adversely affect the grieving process for relatives.

It is often stated that certain groups need to bury their dead in a particular way. While this information is potentially useful, this should not be an opportunity to stereotype people or groups of people who find themselves living away from their place of origin; in individual circumstances the perceptions of a particular person may be extremely variable.

Moreover, the deceased may not wish for their customs to be strictly adhered to, thus it is absolutely necessary to check and verify, wherever possible, what the anticipated plans are, irrespective of cultural group.

Case histories provide a good illustration of this. For example it is stated that a person who is Jewish needs to be buried within hours, in other words preferably on the day of death. In addition a post mortem is disallowed unless there is a legal requirement for this (Fellowes 1995). Some Christians can either be buried or cremated while some can only be buried, and the patient may wish to see a priest before death 'for the last confession'. There is no apparent restriction on a post mortem.

The problem with this type of account is that it is reductionist and in many ways not particularly helpful. It is important to ask whether the Jewish person was 'orthodox', 'liberal' or 'reform', since this will ultimately determine the practices. In the second example it is clearly dependent on what type of Christian, for example the many variants all approach this period after death in different ways. Perhaps most importantly, the deceased may not wish to follow any religious practises and thus much of this discussion becomes invalid. The point behind this is that there is more to culture than merely religion and asking, exploring and discussing is much more useful than assuming.

Grief

'One often calms one's grief by recounting it' – *Polyeucte*, Act 1, Scene 3, Pierre Corneille (1606–84), French dramatist.

It is fairly safe to say that no two people will ever experience grief in the same way; the person who has just died will undoubtedly be unique as is the loved one, partner or friend who 'has been left behind'. This section focuses almost entirely on the person who is bereaved. Some of the feelings which occur in the immediate period following death are fear, helplessness, sadness, longing, guilt, shame and anger. A brief description of each of these will follow.

Fear

Feelings of fear are easy to understand though difficult to 'rationalise' somehow. Fears may arise out of being left alone or of not being able to cope in the period after the burial or the cremation. This is often the most difficult time anyway. It may be that the person who has died was very practical, thus another fear is that the bereaved will have to undertake tasks which have not been done before. Perhaps the most insidious fear is that of breaking down or having a 'nervous breakdown' (see later this chapter and Chapter 5).

Helplessness

Because friends and family often rally around in the immediate period, this feeling of true helplessness does not occur until two or three weeks after the actual death. This may be a feeling or perception of helplessness rather than real helplessness and may be reflective of a loss in confidence or self-esteem.

Sadness

It is inevitable and normal that sadness is felt and experienced in this period. The period of sadness is extremely variable and will depend on many factors such as personality, expectation, culture and many others. The intensity of this sadness is worthy of comment. Some people cannot ever imagine the sadness, which in itself is all-encompassing and pervasive, ever diminishing. While this last point is clearly untrue it reveals the depth of the sadness which can occur in this period after death.

Guilt

Guilt is common and may again depend on many factors, for example, a feeling that the bereaved has outlived the person who has just died. This is particularly common of parents who have seen their children die, almost irrespective of age. Part of the reason for this is that contemporary

Westerners have come to believe that children will outlive their parents. When this is not the case, and HIV infection unfortunately provides a good example, guilt is often a feature of the grief.

Shame

Sometimes the bereaved feel shame for having been emotional at such a time, in other words showing their real need for support and help. It may be that the alternative lifestyle of the deceased comes to be associated with those who have been bereaved, especially if such lifestyles, for example being gay or an injecting drug user, are stigmatised or not wholly accepted by society.

Anger

Anger is another characteristic which points to the senselessness (and perhaps finality) of death. Of course tied in with this are questions about why this should have happened, why now and even why me? Part of this natural questioning process also brings to the fore unresolved queries such as what could have been done to prevent the death. Again this is part of a natural adjustment to what is a normal part of the grieving process. Nevertheless for the bereaved person these feelings do not feel 'normal' at all, and are heightened if they have not encountered death previously.

Box 11.2   Key points about grief for the bereaved

- You are basically the same person that you were before the death.
- There is light at the end of the tunnel.
- There is help available if you feel that you need help with this process.

Memories and hopes

Of course some would argue that memories are the only remnants that are left following the death of a loved one. If that is the case then one strategy is to cherish them, while not allowing them to become the total focus of attention at all times. Memories, especially at the beginning, will be linked with feelings of loss. The bereaved may not wish to dwell on memories for too long because of the pain and other associated feelings which are conjured up.

For health workers this presents an opportunity, especially when following-up with the bereaved. Although not appropriate for all, some clinicians specifically ask the person recently bereaved to bring along a photograph album or 'memory-box' in order to spend some time talking about the person who has died. Often it is possible in these discussions to determine the extent to which the person is adjusting to their new life.

Another idea is to promote the use of a video recording in order to try and cherish the memories for as long as possible. This particular strategy is useful for children. Video recording presents a remarkably adept and accessible way of recording images of a parent, perhaps for when the child is older in order for them to identify with the parent they will not know.

It is perhaps the lost hopes and aspirations which are the most difficult to deal with from the bereaved's point of view. Once again it is entirely normal that the person feels this way, though these negative feelings should recede as time passes. The health care worker is sometimes left feeling that little can be done; however, just being there, listening and acknowledging that these feelings are powerful, real and discomforting is what is important.

Physical and emotional sensations of grief

Along with the feelings mentioned above it is common for the bereaved to suffer with a host of 'bodily symptoms' which range from insomnia, poor appetite, tiredness, 'fuzziness', a lack of concentration, loss of memory, palpitations, dizziness, nausea and diarrhoea, headaches, back pains, generalised aches and pains and abnormal periods. Although these sound very worrying, they are part of what is called an 'anxiety-related' syndrome, in this case secondary to the death of the loved one. In fact they can be likened to similar effects which are suffered in times of any major stress.

First, if the bereaved is experiencing any of these symptoms and feels there is something 'physical' about this condition it is absolutely in order to seek advice from a general practitioner (GP). Not only will the GP then know what has happened but they may be able to help in several different ways.

Second, the GP is in a much better position to clarify whether these wide-ranging symptoms are normal or not. After all, it may be that a new and separate physical problem manifests in the bereavement period. Commonly the bodily symptoms listed above are due to and part and parcel of the bereavement process.

Third, help can be provided to those suffering specific problems; for example a person may be sleeping very badly, and subsequently feels very tired and listless, which is then made worse by the insomnia. It is common practice for GPs to prescribe for this type of scenario, in order to break this cycle of poor sleep and tiredness. The best medications belong to the benzodiazepine group (commonly Valium or Temazepam, see Chapter 8) which are called anxiolytics and reduce anxiety and aid relaxation.

Some people may be very wary of such medications, and this wariness is absolutely right and proper. However, for very short periods, for example four to five days, these medications have a legitimate place in the management of anxiety-related disorders. The real difficulty arises if the same person returns having used up the medication in the allotted time and requests more; it is easy to see that repeat prescriptions could result from the request, which is wrong and inappropriate. The reason for this is that such drugs are easily tolerated and have major addictive potential. While they are fine to use for a few days at a time, for anything longer (as short as two weeks), the person starts to feel withdrawal effects after stopping them.

Help during the bereavement process

It is important to know more about the various feelings and experiences that people articulate around this time.

Numbness

As stated previously numbness is commonly felt in the immediate period. Some refer to this as shock, others as shocked disbelief. Numbness is a protective instinct, shielding the person from the true extent of the loss. It is common for the bereaved who react in this way to be 'abnormally calm', while they themselves report feelings of inner turmoil, mental anguish and even 'unreality'. Moreover the bereaved may feel they are going through the events as if they were a dream, almost as if they were 'watching' these events unravel (this is called 'de-personalisation').

Feelings that the dead person is still present

While this sounds bizarre and unreal, it is very common for the bereaved sometimes to perceive the dead person as being alive, even walking around the house or flat. Sometimes this may be an apparition and can be frightening or reassuring, depending on circumstance and previous beliefs. These experiences can be linked to searching behaviour, in other words the bereaved does not want to believe that death has occurred; usually a degree of denial is normal and protective.

Activities

Activities can present a useful opportunity at this time, although there is a fine line between remaining active and becoming so active that it prevents the help that is so obviously required. This latter phenomena is called 'blocking': while some of this is acceptable and indeed expected, blocking actually prevents the bereaved from adjusting to a life without the deceased if sustained (see later).

Reality

Perhaps one of the more useful activities is to confront reality, in other words attending the funeral, inspecting losses and memory-boxes and watching video recordings if available. This is linked with 'going over the event', almost to the point of reliving the last few days or hours. While this has an element of denial to it – though normal – the need to do this is sometimes real and tangible.

Support

While it is common for people to wish for privacy at such times, it can also be reassuring for some that others are going through this same process. This sharing with others can be an important component of the healing process.

Box 11.3　A basic guide about when to seek help for grief

- If the patient cannot handle such intense feelings, including the bodily sensations. Alternatively, if the period of grief appears prolonged (this unfortunately is extremely difficult to define), or the person continues to feel confused, empty or even exhausted from the recent events.
- Some say that a month is about the time when feelings of emptiness, confusion, numbness start to wane, though once again this is highly variable.
- If night-time dreams and nightmares continue and start to affect the bereaved person during the day, this may be a pointer to accessing further help.
- If the sudden loss has left the bereaved feeling isolated with no real prospect of sharing these feelings with others.
- If the bereaved person is having problems relating to close friends,

---

or new difficulties manifest themselves, such as psycho-sexual problems.
- Accidents are more common and if a person suffers a series of accidents this may be a sign that further help is warranted.
- It is probably not a good sign if the bereaved excessively smokes, drinks or uses drugs in order to try and ameliorate certain feelings towards the event. This is a difficult problem and depends to a large extent on the amount of insight the bereaved has towards these behaviours.
- Related to the last section, if work is suffering from either the bereavement or the effects of drink and drugs, it seems sensible to seek help. Of course work may suffer because the bereaved has returned too quickly (once again, this is hard to define). Perhaps it should be the quality of work which determines overall work performance at this difficult time.

How to differentiate between normal and abnormal in the grieving process?

This is an extremely difficult question and unfortunately cannot really be answered. The point has been made that the process of grief and bereavement is an individualised and often private one which cannot always be neatly described and packaged into something generalisable. However, in stating this, this is very much a Western-style view of bereavement as many will recognise. In other cultures and in other ethnic groups, death is treated in different ways, expectations are different and grief is more of a collective feeling of loss, not so much the individualised feelings which predominate in the UK (Helman 1994).

A recent review of a psychologically-oriented model of the phases of bereavement will be described before exploring deviations from this (Woof and Carter 1997).

Numbing: As stated previously the first and most immediate phase starts with stunned disbelief. Simultaneously there may be anger, anxiety or a combination of all three.

Yearning and searching: Again as described this phase appears after a few days, perhaps even weeks where the bereaved has intense feelings of distress and longing, combined with perceptions of the deceased. At this time there is an endless round of going over and revisiting the last few days or hours, almost to the point of obsession.

Disorganisation and despair: This is the phase, often extending into weeks and months, in which it is clear to the bereaved that previous patterns of behaviour need to change in order to adjust to these new circumstances, in other words as a person who has lost a loved one. Feelings of anger, anxiety and depression can accompany this phase.

Reorganisation: Here there is at last light at the end of the tunnel. The bereaved will have had time to acknowledge the enormity of what has happened; the irreversibility may well still be dawning, but a re-configuration will be taking place. This final phase ought to leave the person actively adjusting to a new phase in their own lives, without forgetting the events of the recent past.

It has already been implied that bereavement is one of the accepted risk factors for clinical depression. Depression following this type of event is said to feel qualitatively different and studies show that it occurs all too commonly. Counselling, psychotherapy or anti-depressants all have their part to play in attempting to reverse these feelings (see Chapter 10 for a further exploration of the use of anti-depressants).

Concentrating on mental health, adults who have been bereaved also show vulnerability to greater anxiety, increased use of prescribed medication and suicide (Woof & Carter 1997). In terms of physical health, a number of studies are inconclusive although some show increased incidence of life-threatening disorders.

Finally, we return to the question of how to differentiate between what is normal and abnormal grieving. These are very difficult to define, and while the extremes may be easy to discern, the more ambiguous areas need more research. General practitioners are a group of clinicians who have traditionally cared for those who have been bereaved, although their exact input remains variable and difficult to quantify. Obviously general support, providing medical certificates and monitoring the progress of the recently bereaved are three areas in which their input are called upon. Whether general practitioners ought to be more consistently involved with such processes is unknown.

Box 11.4   Useful tips about the bereavement process for individuals

- Don't bottle up feelings.
- Don't avoid talking about these experiences.
- Don't expect the memories to fade instantly.
- Do express how you feel, your emotions.

- Do take the opportunity to review the experience.
- Do look after yourself (take time out, rest, sleep).
- Do try to maintain a routine at the beginning, it may help.
- Drive more carefully (accidents are more common at times of major stress).
- Be more careful around the house or flat (for the same reason).
- Don't overlook the children, they have feelings too.
- Do send the children back to school and maintain their activities.
- Do let their teacher know about what has happened.

Bereavement in gay couples

Much of the earlier work in bereavement and grief reactions was undertaken in 'heterosexual couples'. Is there anything special about gay relationships which sets them aside from the heterosexual group? The answer to this is probably not, except that the stigmatisation – which has been a feature of this text throughout – means that gay bereaved individuals are particularly vulnerable to isolation, hostility and potential loss of material wealth if a will had not been made (King 1993).

For example a gay man who is bereaved may not find the sympathy and help he receives on his return to work is the same as someone else who is bereaved but is heterosexual. The reason for this may be simple prejudice or a perception that gay relationships are not as legitimate as heterosexual ones. Studies are appearing which suggest that in the major urban centres of HIV infection and AIDS (New York, San Francisco, London, Amsterdam, Paris) that some individuals have suffered with multiple bereavements (King 1993, Maasen 1998). The bereavement work that needs to be done in such circumstances will be different but no less valid. It is also likely that a specialist counsellor or clinician who is familiar with such syndromes will be available.

Who to consult for help in the period after death?

It will be obvious from this section that many members of the primary care team can be consulted in the period after the death of the loved one. It seems sensible that where the general practitioner has been involved with the person and their carers in the terminal phase of the illness that the doctor can be approached. However, it is not important who the health professional is, so long as they are familiar with the aftermath of what can be a very painful process. As implied above there are other options. While most of these are usually accessible through the general practitioner, some services accept self-referrals.

In larger cities there is often a locality-based bereavement counselling service or the surgery may have their own practice-based counsellor, which can be much more convenient. Large voluntary organisations, perhaps exemplified by the bigger units in London such as the Terence Higgins Trust and London Lighthouse, provide independent counselling services for this type of need (see 'Useful Addresses' at the end of this volume).

Rarely, bereavement results in more serious mental health problems, for example acute anxiety, clinical depression, neurosis and even frank psychosis (see Chapter 5 for a comprehensive description). Perhaps these can be best categorised as conditions which affect the person in such profound ways that their grasp of reality is reduced (psychosis). Alternatively their levels of anxiety, or behaviour indicate that they are functioning so badly that further help is warranted. It is common for this condition to be part of a depression even though the latter is not as obvious as the anxiety. In either condition the mental state of the bereaved may deteriorate to such an extent that suicide is considered and acted upon. For these conditions – which clearly lie at the more serious end of a wide mental health spectrum – a clinician is probably the most appropriate person to approach such as a doctor or nurse-practitioner (see Chapter 5).

References

CRUSE (nd) 'Coping with a major personal crisis (bereavement care)', leaflet produced by CRUSE – Bereavement Care, London.

Fellowes, D. (1995) *Health and Culture: Information File*, London: Health Services and Research Evaluation Unit, Lewisham Hospital Trust.

Helman, C. (1994) *Health, Culture, Health and Illness*, (third edition), London: Butterworth-Heinemann.

King, M. (1993) *AIDS, HIV and Mental Health*, London: Cambridge University Press.

Maasen, T. (1998) 'Counselling gay men with multiple loss and survival problems', *AIDS-CARE* (special issue devoted to the third Home and Community Care conference, May 1997, Amsterdam, The Netherlands), vol. 10, supplement 1: 557–63.

McCrory, P. (1994) 'Dealing with Funerals', leaflet produced by Body Positive, London.

Office of National Statistics (July 1996) 'Death certification and referral to the coroner' (Letter to doctors).

Turner, J. and Raphael, B. (1997) 'Requesting necropsies', *British Medical Journal*, 314: 1499–1500.

Woof, W.R. and Carter, Y. (1997) 'The grieving adult and the general practitioner: a literature review in two parts' (Parts 1 & 2), *British Journal of General Practice*, 47: 443–8 and 509–14.

Useful Addresses

The following is a list of useful addresses and contact numbers.

Black HIV/AIDS Network (BAHN), St Stephens House, 41 Uxbridge Road, London W12 8LH. Telephone: 0181 749 2828.
Provides services in multilingual settings for people with HIV.

Blackliners, Unit 46, Eurolink Centre, 49 Effra Road, London SW2 1BZ. Helpline: 0171 738 5274.
Counselling, care and support for people affected by HIV and AIDS who are African, Asian or Caribbean.

Body Positive, 51b Philbeach Gardens, London SW5 9EB. Helpline: 0171 373 9124.
Provides counselling, self-help groups and support.

Grandmas, PO Box 1392, London SW6E 4EJ. Telephone: 0171 610 3904.
Support for families affected by HIV including babysitting, children's outings and social events.

Haemophilia Society, 123 Westminster Bridge Road, London SE1 7HR. Telephone: 0171 928 2020.

HIV/AIDS Treatment Update/Directory and the National AIDS Manual. Available via NAM publications, 16a Clapham Common, Southside, London SW4 7AB. Telephone: 0171 627 3200.
These publications provide extensive and comprehensive information about treatments, hospital centres, medical tests, new trials, etc.

Immunity Legal Centre, 1st Floor, 32–38 Osnaburgh Street, London NW1 3ND. Telephone: 0171 388 6776.
Legal advice centre for people with HIV and AIDS.

Landmark, 47 Tulse Hill, London SW2 2TN. Telephone: 0181 678 6686.
A centre for people with HIV which offers various therapies, advice and counselling.

London Lighthouse, 111–117 Lancaster Road, London W11 1QT. Telephone: 0171 792 1200.
Residential and support groups for people with HIV infection.

Mainliners, 205 Stockwell Road, London SW9 9SL. Telephone: 0171 737 3141.
Service for people who are drug users affected by HIV.

Mildmay Mission Hospital, Hackney Road, London E2 7NA. Telephone: 0171 739 2331.
Residential care for people with HIV.

MIND: National Association for Mental Health, Granta House, Broadway, London E15 4BQ. Telephone: 0181 519 2122.

National AIDS Helpline 0800 567123 (24 hour).

Positive Options, 22 Angel Gate, London EC1V 2PT. Telephone: 0171 278 5039.
This offers advice on planning the future, particularly for families and children with HIV.

Positively Women, 5 Sebastian Street, London EC1V 0HE. Helpline: 0171 490 2327.
Support services for women with HIV infection.

Refugee Council, Bondway House, 3–9 Bondway, London SW8 1SJ. Telephone: 0171 820 3000.
Offers advice for refugees and asylum seekers.

SANE, Cityside House, 40 Adler Street, London E1 1EE. SANE-line: 0345 678000.
Formerly 'Schizophrenia: A National Emergency', now open to all mental health problems.

Terence Higgins Trust, 52–54 Grays Inn Road, London WC1X 8JU. Helpline: 0171 242 1010.

Libraries

- Many local public libraries will have sections on HIV/AIDS.
- The Terence Higgins Trust library has detailed information, newsletters, journals, etc. Telephone: 0171 831 0330 for further information.
- Body Positive (London) has an information room. Telephone: 0171 835 1045.
- Crusaid information exchange provides information via computer based at the Chelsea and Westminster Hospital, 369 Fulham Rd, SW10 9NH.

Glossary

AIDS – Acquired Immune Deficiency Syndrome. Defined as a condition whereby depletion of T4 lymphocytes by the HIV virus causes a significant opportunistic infection or AIDS-defining illness.

Anti-virals – Drugs which are used to fight viral infection, often generically used to describe drugs fighting HIV infection.

Combination therapies – The use of two, three or four anti-viral drugs used simultaneously to fight HIV infection.

HAART – Highly active antiretroviral therapy, refers to use of combination anti-viral treatment. Usually three anti-viral drugs.

HIV – Human immuno-deficiency virus, which causes depletion of a particular subset of white blood cells (CD4 or T cell lymphocytes).

Immuno-suppression – The reduced ability of the immune system to cope with infection.

Opportunistic disease – Diseases which primarily affect people with weakened immune systems.

Protease – The enzyme which breaks proteins into smaller sections. Protease inhibitors are drugs which stop this and so prevent HIV replication.

Post-exposure prophylaxis - Anti-viral treatment that is given to someone (usually health care workers) following a needle-stick injury or accident at work.

Retrovirus – The family of viruses to which HIV belongs.

Reverse transcriptase – The enzyme that is essential to convert RNA to DNA to enable HIV to replicate successfully.

Seroconversion (primary HIV infection) – Flu-like illness that approximately 60 per cent of people will experience a few weeks after exposure to HIV.

T cells (CD4 cells) – The cells that the HIV virus primarily infects and depletes. These are part of the lymphocyte sub-section of white blood cells which fight infection.

Viral load – A test whereby the amount of virus present in a blood sample can be estimated. Useful as a prognostic marker and as a measure of how effective anti-viral treatments are.

Vertical transmission – This refers to transmission (of HIV) from mother to baby.

Window period – This refers to the three-month period following exposure to HIV during which it takes full antibody production to occur. During this time an HIV test may be positive, negative or equivocal.

Further Reading

Adler, M.W. (1991) *The ABC of AIDS*, Second edition, London: British Medical Association Press.

Anderson W. and Weatherburn, P. (1996) *The treatment information needs of people living with HIV*, London: NAM Publications.

Barter, G., Barton, S. and Gazzard, B. (1993) *HIV and AIDS – Your questions answered*, Edinburgh: Churchill-Livingstone.

Beiser, C. (1997) 'HIV infection-2', *British Medical Journal*, 314: 579–583.

Beaumont, B. (1997) *Care of drug-users in General Practice*, Oxford: Radcliffe Press.

Boyd, K.M., Higgs, R. and Pinching, A.J. (1997) *The new dictionary of Medical Ethics*, London: BMJ Publishing Group.

Cohen, P.T., Sande, M.A. and Volberding, P.A. (1990) *The AIDS knowledge base*: a textbook on HIV disease from the University of California, San Francisco, and the San Francisco General Hospital, Massachusetts: The Medical Press.

Communicable Disease Report (1997) 'The epidemiology of HIV infection and AIDS', *CDR*, Vol. 7 (review no. 9), August.

Cohn, J.A. (1997) 'HIV infection-1', *British Medical Journal*, 314: 487–91.

Curtis, H. and Hoolaghan, Jewitt C. (1995) *Sexual health promotion in general practice*, Oxford: Radcliffe Medical Press.

Croser, D., Erridge, P. and Robinson, P. (1994) *HIV and Dentistry*, British Dental Association (BDA) Occasional Paper No. 4.

Cusack, L. and Singh, S. (eds) (1994) *HIV and AIDS Care – practical approaches*, London: Chapman and Hall.

Department of Health (1997) 'Unlinked Anonymous HIV Prevalence Monitoring Programme, England and Wales', London: Department of Health.

Drugs and Therapeutics Bulletin (1997) 'Major advances in the treatment of HIV-1 infection', 35: No. 4, April.

Haughton, N. (1997) *Management of HIV/AIDS in general practice*, London: BMA Foundation for AIDS.

King, M. (1993) *AIDS, HIV and Mental Health*, Cambridge: Cambridge University Press.

Levy, L. (1997) 'A guide to good practice for sexual health promotion and HIV prevention in primary care settings', London: Lambeth, Southwark and Lewisham Health Authority and The HIV project.

OHE (Office of Health Economics) (1991) 'Dying with dignity', No. 97 in a series of reports about health problems, London.

Madge, S. and Singh, S. (1998) 'The new imperative to test for HIV in pregnancy', *British Journal of General Practice*, 48: 1127–8.

Main, J., Moyle, G., Peters, B. and Coker, R. (1995) *What we should all know about HIV & AIDS*, London: Mediscript Ltd.

Matthews, P. (1994) *HIV disease – a guide for GPs with HIV positive patients*, Birmingham: Birmingham Health Authority.

Mann, Jonathan (1992) 'AIDS in the 1990s: A Global analysis', Malcom Morris Memorial Lecture, *Journal of the Royal Society of Health*, 112(3), June.

Mansfield, S. and Singh, S. (1990) *The management of HIV/AIDS in primary care*, London: BMA Foundation for AIDS.

Miller, D., Weber, J. and Green, J. (1986) *The management of AIDS patients*, London: MacMillan Press.

Miller, R. and Murray, D. (1998) *HIV and social work – Practitioner's Guide*, Birmingham: Venture Press.

Moss, A. (1992) *HIV and AIDS: Management by the primary care team*, Oxford: Oxford University Press.

NAM (1996) *National AIDS Manual/AIDS directory: a directory of a range of services*, London: NAM Publications.

Regnaud, C. and Davies, A. (1986) *A guide to symptom relief in advanced cancer*, fourth edition, Manchester: Books for Midwives Press.

Richardson, A. and Bolle, D. (1992) *Wise before their time: people with AIDS and HIV talk about their lives*, London: Fount Harper-Collins.

Schlyter, C. (1992) *Advance directives & AIDS: an empirical study of the interest in living wills and proxy decision making in the context of HIV/AIDS care*, London: Centre of Medical Law and Ethics.

Shaw, M., Tomlinson, D. and Higginson, I. (1996) 'Survey of HIV patients' views on confidentiality and non-discrimination policies in General practice', *British Medical Journal*, 312: 1463–4.

Sherr, L. (ed.) (1997) *AIDS and Adolescents*, Amsterdam, The Netherlands: Harwood Academic Publications.

Sherr, L. and van den Boom, F. (1995) 'AIDS and suicide', *AIDS-CARE*, special issue, vol. 7, supplement 2.

Sims, R. and Moss, V. (1991) *Terminal care for people with AIDS*, London: Edward Arnold Publishers.

Singh, S., Wigersma, L. and van den Boom, F. (1998) 'The 3rd International Conference on Home and Community Care for Persons Living with HIV/AIDS', *AIDS-CARE*, special issue, vol. 10, supplement 1.

Smith, S., Robinson, J. Hollyer et al. (1996) 'Combining specialist and primary health care teams for HIV positive patients: retrospective and prospective studies', *British Medical Journal*, 312: 416–20.

Starace, F. and Sherr, L. (1998) 'Suicidal behaviours, euthanasia and AIDS', *AIDS* (In press).

Twycross, R. (1997) *Introducing Palliative Care*, Oxford: Radcliffe Medical Press.

UNAIDS (1996) 'The right to care', Bulletin from the Joint United Nations Programme on HIV/AIDS, Geneva: UNAIDS.

Williams, I, Mindel, A. and Weller, I. (1989) *AIDS pocket picture guides*, London: Gower Medical Publishing.

Youle, M., Clarbour, J., Wade, P. and Farthing, C. (1988), *AIDS Therapeutics in HIV Disease*, Edinburgh: Churchill-Livingstone.

Index